HEAL YOURSELF
Naturally

HEAL YOURSELF
Naturally

Safe, Effective Treatment Plans as Featured in *Health Counselor* Magazine

Edited by
Karolyn A. Gazella

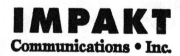

IMPAKT
Communications • Inc.

Heal Yourself
Naturally

Safe, Effective Treatment Plans
as featured in *Health Counselor* magazine

Edited by
Karolyn A. Gazella

Copyright © 1996 IMPAKT Communications, Inc.
Library of Congress Catalog Card Number: 96-75574
ISBN 0-9647489-2-4

Cover design by Archetype Group

To order contact:
IMPAKT Communications, Inc.
P.O. Box 12496
Green Bay, WI 54307-2496
Credit card orders can call 1-800-477-2995
FAX (414) 499-3441
Quantity discounts are available.

Dedication

This book is dedicated to the loving memory of Eunice Gazella as she continues to touch our lives and help us with our journey.

And to all of the loyal readers of *Health Counselor* magazine and those who read this book. May you discover good health, peace, and happiness. Live your life with passion and you will be fulfilled.

Contents

Foreword. X

Acknowledgements XI

Preface XII

Introduction 1

Acne. 7

Age Spots 9

AIDS and HIV Infection 10

Alcoholism 13

Alzheimer's Disease, Senility, and Dementia 16

Anemia. 18

Angina 19

Ankylosing Spondylitis (see Rheumatoid Arthritis) 23

Anxiety. 23

Arthritis (see Gout, Osteoarthritis, or Rheumatoid Arthritis) 24

Arrhythmias (see Angina) 24

Asthma 25

Atherosclerosis (see Cholesterol). 26

Attention Deficit Disorder 27

Bladder Infections 31

Blood Clots (see Thrombophlebitis). 32

Boils. 32

Bone Spurs 33

Bronchitis and Pneumonia 34

Bruises 35

Bursitis and Tendonitis 37

Cancer 38

Candidiasis 41

Canker Sores 47

Carpal Tunnel Syndrome 48

Cataracts 49

Cellulite 50

Cerebrovascular Insufficiency 51

Chemotherapy (see Cancer) 53

Cholesterol, Elevated Blood Levels 53

Chronic Fatigue Syndrome 55

Cold Sores 57

Common Cold 58

Colitis (see Crohn's Disease and Ulcerative Colitis) 59

Constipation 59

Crohn's Disease and Ulcerative Colitis 61

Depression 62

Dermatitis (see Eczema) 64

Detoxification 64

Diabetes 65

Ear Infections and Chronic Otitis Media 68

Eczema 70

Endometriosis 71

Fibroid (Uterine) 72

Fibrocystic Breast Disease 73

Food Allergy 75

Gallstones 77

Glaucoma 78

Gout 80

Hair and Skin 81

Hayfever (see Asthma) 82

Headache (also see Migraine) 82

Heart Disease (see Cholesterol or Angina). 83

Hemorrhoids. 83

Hepatitis 85

Herpes 87

Hiatal Hernia 89

High Blood Pressure 89

Hives 91

Hot Flashes (see Menopause). 92

Hyperactivity (see Attention Deficit Disorder) 92

Hypoglycemia. 92

Hypothyroidism. 93

Impotence. 95

Indigestion 97

Infections 100

Infertility (Female) 101

Infertility (Male). 102

Insomnia. 104

Irritable Bowel Syndrome. 105

Kidney Stones 106

Lupus 107

Lyme Disease 109

Macular Degeneration 110

Menopause 111

Menstrual Disorders
(see appropriate topic, e.g., Infertility, Fibrocystic Breast Disease, PMS) . 113

Migraine Headache. 113

Mononucleosis (see Infections). 115

Multiple Sclerosis 115

Osteoarthritis. 117

Osteoporosis 120

Parasites (Intestinal) 124

Parkinson's Disease 125

Peridontal Disease and Gingivitis 127

Pleurisy (see Bronchitis and Pneumonia) 129

Premenstrual Syndrome 129

Prostate Enlargement (BPH) 130

Prostatitis 132

Psoriasis 134

Rheumatoid Arthritis 135

Rosacea 138

Schizophrenia and Multiple Personality Disorder 139

Scleroderma 140

Sinus Infection 142

Sports Injuries (see Bursitis and Tendonitis) 143

Stress 143

Strokes (see Cerebrovascular Insufficiency) 145

Sore Throat and Tonsillitis (see Infections) 145

Surgery Preparation and Recovery 148

Ulcer 149

Varicose Veins 150

Weight Loss 151

Appendix I (Quick Reference Guide to Nutrients) 155

Appendix II (Quick Reference Guide to Herbal Extracts) 163

Appendix III (Health Counselor Index) 171

Appendix IV (Book listing) 187

Glossary 190

Sidebar Index 193

Foreword

In our journey to protect our health and the health of those we love, we are bombarded by information that can be confusing and sometimes inaccurate.

Health Counselor magazine has been giving the gift of valuable information to readers for more than eight years. Some of the finest healthcare professionals in the world have contributed their knowledge and expertise to *Health Counselor* magazine. *Heal Yourself Naturally* is a compilation of that hard work and dedication.

This book is a prime example of dependable information taken from highly reputable sources and presented in an easy-to-read, understandable format. It is an extremely valuable reference that will be an important addition to your natural health library.

Within the pages of this book, you will find practical treatment plans for a wide variety of illnesses. The information is concise and the recommendations are valuable. This book follows my belief that it is important to look beyond merely curing the obvious symptoms. We need to look for the cause of the illness and find a cure for that source. In order to do this we must take a comprehensive approach that involves diet, nutritional supplements, mind/body concepts, exercise, and spirituality. This book provides sound advice regarding diet and nutritional supplements, two very valuable components to any successful healthcare plan.

A truly successful health program begins and ends with education and accurate information. *Heal Yourself Naturally* will prove to be an important addition to your natural health knowledge. The recommendations and treatment ideas will help you gain better health while assisting you physically, emotionally, and financially.

My congratulations to Karolyn Gazella and the entire *Health Counselor* staff on a job well-done.

Dr. Jan de Vries

Acknowledgements

This book would not be possible without the assistance and dedication of the many healthcare professionals who write for *Health Counselor* magazine. These individuals should be complimented not only for the valuable information they provide, but also the work they do in their private practices, writing books, lecturing, teaching, and educating people about the many benefits of natural medicine. The talented contributing authors of *Health Counselor* magazine are: Kevon Arthurs, N.D.; Judy L. Christianson, N.D.; Anthony J. Cichoke, D.C.; Carolyn DeMarco, M.D.; Alan Gaby, M.D.; Ann Louise Gittleman; Siri Khalsa; Patrick Quillin, Ph.D., R.D., C.N.S.; Jan McBarron, M.D.; Alexander Schauss, Ph.D.; Charles B. Simone, M.D.; and Jonathan V. Wright, M.D.

A very special thanks to Michael T. Murray, N.D., who is a long-standing contributing author of *Health Counselor* magazine and the editor of *The American Journal of Natural Medicine*, also published by IMPAKT Communications, Inc. Also to Frances FitzGerald, an extremely talented health writer who has been featured in *Health Counselor* extensively.

Of course, heartfelt appreciation to the entire IMPAKT staff: Kathi Magee, vice president and administrative coordinator; Shelly Petska, sales and marketing director; Lisa Nischke, distribution assistant; and Maria Konkel, executive assistant. Your dedication and hard work does not go unnoticed.

To all of the manufacturers of quality products, especially Enzymatic Therapy, Inc., one of the finest supplement companies in the industry. Thank you for your commitment to producing products that work.

And finally, to all of the independent health food store owners and their employees—what a valuable, wonderful service you provide!

Preface

Before you read on...

- Do not self-diagnose. Proper medical care is critical to good health. If you have symptoms suggestive of an illness discussed in this book, please consult a physician, preferably a naturopathic doctor (N.D.), holistic M.D. or osteopath (D.O.), chiropractor, or other natural healthcare specialist.

- If you are currently on a prescription medicine, you absolutely must work with your doctor before discontinuing any drug. Discontinuing a prescription without medical supervision can be life-threatening.

- If you wish to try the natural approach, discuss it with your physician. Since your physician may be unaware of the natural alternatives available, you may need to educate him/her. Many of the natural products being recommended are based upon published studies in medical journals.

- Remember, although many natural alternatives, such as nutritional supplements and herbs, are effective on their own, they work even better if they are part of a comprehensive natural treatment plan which focuses on diet and lifestyle factors. Do not underestimate the value of a healthy diet and lifestyle.

How to use this book

This book features suggested treatment plans featuring specific nutritional supplements; however, it is important to remember that they are only one aspect of health promotion. Maintaining a positive mental attitude, eating a healthful diet, and regular exercise are critical to achieve and maintain good health.

For your convenience, product recommendations are listed in order of their importance. For further guidance in choosing only some of the products listed, consult with your health food store or natural health provider.

The basic outline for the conditions discussed in this book is as follows:

Description:

This section provides a description and information about the condition.

Dietary and Lifestyle Recommendations:

This section lists important dietary and lifestyle considerations. The general recommendations are to:

1. Consume a diet which focuses on whole, unprocessed foods (whole grains, legumes, vegetables, fruits, nuts, and seeds).
2. Eliminate the intake of alcohol, caffeine, and sugar.
3. Identify and control food allergies.
4. Get regular exercise.
5. Perform a relaxation exercise (deep breathing, meditation, prayer, visualization, etc.) for 10 to 15 minutes each day.
6. Drink at least 48 ounces of water daily.

Primary treatment plan:

The supplement protocols given in this section are designed to provide results. Only the highest quality manufacturers and products are mentioned in this section.

You will notice that for most health conditions discussed in this section, the following supplements will be recommended:

Doctor's Choice (either for men or women) (Enzymatic Therapy)
    One tablet three times daily.
Doctor's Choice Antioxidant Complex (Enzymatic Therapy)
    One to two tablets three times daily.
Doctor's Choice Flax Oil Plus (Enzymatic Therapy)
    One tablespoon daily.

These formulas serve as a strong foundation upon which to build an effective supplementation protocol. A quality multivitamin mineral formula, comprehensive antioxidant formula, and flax oil will provide you with the necessary nutrients to get on the road to good health.

Additional Recommendations:

This section provides additional information to consider. Usually these recommendations are to be utilized if there is little or no response to the previous recommendations.

Comments:

This section provides interesting facts, warnings, and general information on the entire protocol given for a particular health condition.

Product Recommendations

It has always been the policy of *Health Counselor* magazine to avoid making specific product recommendations. Over the years, we have received countless calls and letters asking what we would recommend specifically for a particular condition. So, with this book, we've decided to bend the rules a bit. After the particular nutritional supplement, herb, or formulation recommended, we have featured the manufacturer of that product in parentheses.

Our product recommendations come from very reliable sources and feature manufacturers we are proud to be associated with. To assist you with information regarding the products listed, here is more information about the key manufacturers featured in this book:

Alta Health Products = 1-800-423-4155 or 1-818-796-1047 (CA)

Barlean's = 1-800-445-3529

BioForce = 1-800-645-9135

Carlson Labs = 1-800-323-4141

Enzymatic Therapy = 1-800-783-2286

Flora = 1-800-498-3610

Natrol = 1-800-326-1520

Keep in mind that the products mentioned in this book are only suggestions. Your local health food store can provide you with more information and direction.

Introduction

Over the past eight years, *Health Counselor* magazine has been educating the American public about natural medicine. We've reached millions of people and have been fortunate to work with some of the finest natural healthcare researchers and providers in the United States and Canada. It has always been our mission to bring our readers cutting edge information on how they can prevent and treat illness using natural medicine concepts, products, and services.

This book is a reflection of that commitment. In it we provide practical advice about specific health conditions. Its goal is to give you information you need about natural medicine alternatives. Taking advantage of these suggestions is your choice. And that's the way it should be. You are in charge of your health and your body. It's up to you to get as much information about your particular condition(s) as possible. From there you need to evaluate your options and choose what's best for you. That's the way healthcare was meant to be delivered—with the patient in mind and the patient in control. Doctors, nurses, pharmacists, and health food stores are all sources of information that can provide you with valuable details about options that are available. The rest is up to you!

For your convenience we have also featured a *Health Counselor* cross reference guide in the back of this book. More in-depth information on the condition is featured in the magazine issue listed. To receive a copy of the magazine with the article you are interested in, simply call the toll-free number provided.

What is natural medicine?

It's been called many things: Alternative; holistic; complementary; comprehensive; and yes, even quackery. Even the term "natural medicine" is too limiting, because it is more complex than simply "medicine." It's a philosophy that involves many variables.

Natural medicine is an umbrella term representing a variety of services, products, and treatments. Everything from dietary changes to detoxification procedures can be called holistic and fall into the category of natural medicine. This book will concentrate specifically on nutritional supplements and homeopathic formulas—important aspects of natural medicine. For each condition, dietary and lifestyle recommendations are also provided.

Keep in mind that there are no magic bullets. Health and illness is a very complicated process that requires a comprehensive approach to treatment. Nutritional and homeopathic formulas can provide an important part of any health treatment plan. And that's why so many Americans are drawn to natural medicine.

The natural medicine philosophy believes that the least toxic route should be taken first whenever possible. Nutritional and homeopathic formulas are safe and effective alternatives.

The natural medicine philosophy believes that the power to heal lies within the human body. If you provide your body with the proper tools, it can and will heal itself. Nutritional supplements and homeopathy are ideal tools you can use to support and stimulate the body's healing power. Drugs and surgery are important but should only be used when the body is experiencing a crisis and cannot defend itself properly. Natural medicine looks less at symptoms and more at what is causing the symptoms in the first place. By treating the actual cause, natural medicine provides a long-term solution to short-term symptoms.

What is homeopathy?

Homeopathic medicine has a long-standing history in the United States and Europe. Within the past decade there has been an escalated interest in homeopathy due to the excellent results achieved with little or no toxicity. Homeopathy is a highly individualized form of medicine that works with each person's unique body chemistry.

Homeopathic remedies contain one or more highly diluted natural ingredient(s) that would normally cause the same symptoms of the condition if given in large dosages. It can be compared to a vaccine in that the formula stimulates the body's immune system to fight off the illness.

Because the active component of homeopathic formulas are so diluted (oftentimes, not even detectable through current scientific methods), some conventional medical practitioners reject homeopathy. However, homeopathy not only has a long history of use, it is also supported by many clinical studies. In 1992, the *British Medical Journal* conducted an evaluation of 22 well-designed scientific studies and found that 15 of the 22 showed positive results, indicating that homeopathy provides therapeutic benefits to those who use the formulations. Although homeopathy still remains controversial with some healthcare professionals, positive clinical studies have also been published in other respected journals such as *The Lancet.*

Homeopathy can be used for acute or chronic illnesses as well as for prevention and health promotion purposes. Homeopathic formulas contain naturally occurring plant, animal, or mineral substances and are typically available over-the-counter.

How to use natural medicine

Whether you are a natural medicine novice or a veteran, choosing the right nutritional supplements and homeopathic products can be confusing. The field of natural medicine is constantly expanding and changing to meet the growing needs of the American public. That can make it difficult to stay abreast of what's new in the industry.

That's where your local health food store will be an extremely valuable resource. Health food stores are filled with information and knowledgeable people. Hundreds of health food stores throughout the United States and Canada give away *Health Counselor* magazine as a gift to their loyal shoppers. That shows how committed these stores are to education and information.

Health Counselor is a full-color, 60 to 64 page magazine. With only 20 percent advertising, the focus is on unbiased, accurate editorial. Other natural health publications feature as much as 80 percent advertising and only 20 percent editorial. So, the next time you are visiting your local health food store, ask for *Health Counselor* magazine. *Health Counselor* is also available by subscription (see back of book for ordering details).

If you are interested in finding a natural health provider, contact one of these organizations:

- American Association of Acupuncture and Oriental Medicine
  433 Front St.
  Catasaugua, PA 18032
  (610) 266-1433 FAX (610) 2768

- American Association of Naturopathic Physicians
  2366 Eastlake Ave. East, Suite 322
  Seattle, WA 98102
  (206) 323-7610 Referral Line

- The American Osteopathic Association
  142 E. Ontario St.
  Chicago, IL 60611
  (800) 621-1773

- The American Board of Chelation Therapy
  1407-B North Wells
  Chicago, IL 60610
  (800) 356-2228 FAX (312) 266-3685

- The American Chiropractic Association
  1701 Clarendon Blvd.
  Arlington, VA 22209
  (800) 368-3083

- The American College for Advancement in Medicine
  P.O. Box 3427
  Laguna Hills, CA 92654
  (800) 532-3688 outside CA; (714) 583-7666 CA only

- National Center for Homeopathy
  801 North Fairfax, Suite 306
  Alexandria, VA 22314
  (703) 548-7790

If you are confused about how to get started using natural medicines, your health food store is also filled with great books and information. In addition, there is a list of books available through IMPAKT Communications featured at the back of this book. Here are some general guidelines to follow when purchasing nutritional supplements:

- Always become familiar with the label, knowing exactly what you are taking.
- If you feel uneasy about anything involving the product you are considering, don't take it.
- Always clarify how much you should be taking for your particular circumstance; it's good to clarify this as sometimes you will need to take more or less of a product, depending upon your condition.

- Use products that are guaranteed and shop at stores that stand behind what they sell.
- Get as much information as possible.
- Shop for quality, not cost—remember you're dealing with your health!

For your convenience, all of the products recommended in this book are available at your local health food store. Good luck and remember, optimum health begins with you!

ACNE

Acne is a condition that affects the pores of the skin. A skin pore consists of a canal through which a hair follicle passes. Glands known as sebaceous glands produce sebum, a mixture of oils and waxes, which lubricate the skin and prevent the loss of water. Sebaceous glands are found in highest concentrations on the face, and on the back, chest, and shoulders. Acne affects the areas of the skin that have sebaceous glands.

Acne occurs in two forms: acne vulgaris—affecting the hair follicles and oil-secreting glands of the skin and manifesting as blackheads, whiteheads, and inflammation; and acne conglobata—a more severe form, with deep cyst formation and subsequent scarring.

Acne is most common at puberty due to increased levels of the male sex hormone, testosterone. Although men have higher levels of testosterone than women, during puberty there is an increase of testosterone in both sexes, making girls just as susceptible to acne in this age group. Testosterone causes the sebaceous glands to enlarge and produce more sebum. In addition, the cells that line the skin pore produce more keratin. The combination of increased secretion of sebum and keratin can lead to a blockage of the pore and the formation of a blackhead. With the blockage, bacteria are allowed to overgrow and release enzymes which break down sebum and promote inflammation. This forms what is known as a whitehead or pimple.

To successfully treat acne, a number of dietary and lifestyle factors must be considered. It is also important to support internal body functions, particularly the liver.

Dietary and Lifestyle Recommendations:

- Eliminate all refined and/or concentrated sugars from the diet.
- Do not eat foods containing trans-fatty acids such as milk, milk products, margarine, shortening and other synthetically hydrogenated vegetable oils, as well as fried foods.
- Avoid milk and foods high in iodized salt.
- Avoid the use of greasy creams or cosmetics.
- Wash pillowcases regularly in chemical-free (no added colors or fragrances) detergents.

Primary Treatment Plan:

- Doctor's Choice (Male/Female) (Enzymatic Therapy)
    One tablet three times daily with meals.
- Doctor's Choice Antioxidant Complex (Enzymatic Therapy)
    One capsule three times daily with meals.
- Doctor's Choice Flax Oil Plus (Enzymatic Therapy) or Omega Twin (Barlean's)
    One tablespoon daily.
- Akne-Zyme (Enzymatic Therapy)
    One capsule twice daily.
- Akne Treatment Cream (Enzymatic Therapy)
    Apply one to three times daily as directed.

Additional Recommendations:

- Akne Treatment Cleanser (Enzymatic Therapy)
    Wash face or affected area with the cleanser twice daily.
- Clear Skin (Lehning Laboratories—Homeopathic)
    As directed.
- Lipozyme (Enzymatic Therapy)
    Two to four tablets 20 minutes before meals.
    (Especially beneficial for rosacea and cystic acne.)
- Lympho-Clear (Enzymatic Therapy)
    One capsule three times daily.
- Silymarin (Enzymatic Therapy or Nature's Herbs)
    To support the liver. As directed.
- For adult acne, try Derma Complex (Rainbow Light)
    As directed.

Comments:

Do not use Akne-Zyme during pregnancy (use with caution in women of child-bearing age) or when abdominal pain, nausea or vomiting are present. Akne-Zyme may cause temporary gas.

AGE SPOTS

Age spots are caused by an accumulation of cellular debris known as lipofuscin within cells. In the skin, the lipofuscin deposits can coalesce or clump together to produce brown spots commonly referred to as "age spots." This process is occurring throughout the body, it is just that the skin is all that we see. Typically the cellular debris in a lipofuscin deposit is composed primarily of molecules that have been partially destroyed by free radical damage. The number and severity of age spots are a good indication of the level of oxidative damage that has occurred throughout the body.

Dietary and Lifestyle Recommendations:

- Avoid excessive sun exposure and use sun block creams when in the sun.
- Avoid cigarette smoke, fried foods, and other sources of free radicals.
- Consume a diet rich in plant foods, especially high carotene foods (green leafy vegetables, carrots, yams, sweet potatoes, etc.).
- Drink at least 48 ounces of water daily.

Primary Treatment Plan:

- Doctor's Choice (Male/Female) (Enzymatic Therapy)
      One tablet three times daily.
- Doctor's Choice Antioxidant Complex (Enzymatic Therapy)
      One or two capsules three times daily.
- Carotene Complex (Enzymatic Therapy)
      One or two capsules daily.
- Ginkgo Phytosome (Enzymatic Therapy)
      One capsule two to three times daily.

Additional Recommendations:

- Grape Seed (PCO) Phytosome (Enzymatic Therapy)
      One capsule two to three times daily.
- Beta Carotene (Schiff or Carlson Labs)
      25,000 IU daily.
- Caster Oil topical packs (Home Health or Heritage)
      As directed.

Comments:

Age spots are indicative of free radical and oxidative damage internally as well as on the skin. Julian Whitaker, M.D., recommends a product called Imedeen (Scandinavian Naturals). Imedeen is composed of a special protein and glycosaminoglycan concentrate from fish. Several clinical studies have shown that Imedeen, at an oral dose of 380 to 500 mg daily, can significantly improve the health of the skin and help the skin look younger. Also, when a cosmetic effect is desired, Dr. Whitaker recommends the bleaching agent hydroquinone. Reviva Brown Spot Cream is a popular brand.

AIDS and HIV INFECTION

AIDS (acquired immune deficiency syndrome) is a severe immune deficiency state due to an infection of the human immunodeficiency virus (HIV). The major methods of transmission of HIV are sexual contact, blood to blood contact (through blood transfusions or needle-sharing in drug addicts), and from woman to fetus.

AIDS is not present in all persons infected with HIV. AIDS represents the end stage of the infection and severe depression of the immune system. The goal is to prevent the progression of the disease by supporting the immune system and inhibiting or slowing down the replication of the virus. The dosages given below are most suitable for HIV-positive patients not demonstrating AIDS.

Dietary and Lifestyle Recommendations:

• Do not have unprotected sexual intercourse with persons known or suspected of having HIV or who use intravenous drugs.
• Practice safe sex.
• Do not share a toothbrush, razor, or other implement that could become contaminated with blood from someone with an HIV infection.
• Consume a diet which focuses on whole, unprocessed foods (whole grains, legumes, vegetables, fruits, nuts, and seeds).

(Continued on page 12)

AIDS Update:
High nutrient intake slows disease development.

Certain nutrients, taken in moderate to large doses, can slow the onset of full-blown AIDS in HIV-positive men. That's the conclusion of a study conducted by researchers at The Johns Hopkins Medical Institution in Maryland.

The six-year study, which was published in the December 1993 issue of the *American Journal of Epidemiology*, found that larger amounts of vitamins A, C, B1, and niacin helped HIV-positive men remain free of AIDS for a significantly longer time than individuals taking smaller amounts of these nutrients. Of the 281 men participating in the study:

- Those who had a daily intake of more than 715 mg of vitamin C, 71.4 percent remained AIDS-free, while those who took less than 715 mg of vitamin C per day, only 58.3 percent remained AIDS-free during the study.
- Those who took more than 61 mg per day of niacin, 74.3 percent remained AIDS-free compared to 57.3 percent among those who took less than 61 mg daily of niacin.
- Those who had an intake of between 9,000 IU and 20,000 IU of vitamin A from food sources and supplements had a 45 percent decreased rate of AIDS progression; dosages above 20,000 seemed to actually diminish the effectiveness of this nutrient; well over 75 percent of the men in the study consumed over 180 percent of the Recommended Daily Allowance for vitamin A.
- Those who had a daily intake of over 4.9 mg of vitamin B1 also showed a significant slowed progression of AIDS.

The study also discovered that over 15 mg of zinc taken daily was actually associated with an increased risk of developing full-blown AIDS in HIV-positive patients. The researchers concluded that vitamins A, C, B1, and niacin are important nutrients that can actually help slow the progression of developing full-blown AIDS for HIV-positive individuals.

"The effect we saw was quite substantial—a 40 percent to 48 percent decrease in new AIDS cases in this group that was sustained for more than six years," reported Alice M. Tang, M.S., the study's lead author. "If these results are confirmed by additional studies, we may have a useful intervention for HIV-positive patients."

The researchers concluded that nutrient intake must last for a minimum of two years to realize the benefit, and they recommend HIV-positive individuals start taking these nutrients as soon as possible.

—Johns Hopkins Hospital School of Medicine, Office of Public Affairs; *American Journal of Epidemiology*, Vol. 138, No. 11, 1993.

- Consume adequate protein (consider supplementation with a high quality whey protein at a dosage of 1 gram per 2 pounds body weight).
- Perform a relaxation exercise (deep breathing, meditation, prayer, visualization, etc.) for 10 to 15 minutes each day.
- Get regular exercise (nonstrenuous walking, Tai Chi, stretching, etc.).
- Eliminate the intake of alcohol, caffeine, and sugar.
- Identify and control food allergies.
- Drink at least 48 ounces of water daily.

Primary Treatment Plan:

- Doctor's Choice (Male/Female) (Enzymatic Therapy)
    One tablet three times daily.
- Doctor's Choice Antioxidant Complex (Enzymatic Therapy)
    One to two tablets three times daily.
- Doctor's Choice Flax Oil Plus (Enzymatic Therapy) or Omega Twin (Barlean's)
    One tablespoon daily.
- Vitamin C (any leading brand)
    3,000 to 12,000 mg per day.
- Thymulus (Enzymatic Therapy)
    Two capsules twice daily before meals.
- Carotene Complex (Enzymatic Therapy)
    Four to six capsules daily.
- Mega-Zyme (Enzymatic Therapy)
    Two to four tablets three times daily between meals.

Additional Recommendations:

- A high quality whey protein (Designer Protein) at a dosage of 1 gram per 2 pounds body weight should be used in patients showing signs of muscle wasting or weight loss.
- Cat's Claw (Rainforest Botanicals or Nature's Herbs)
    As directed.
- If liquids are preferred, use Liquid Antioxidant (Natrol).
    As directed.

Comments:

There is concern over the use of echinacea in patients with HIV and AIDS. Although AIDS is associated with wide-spread depression of the immune system and echinacea can dramatically improve immune function in people with low immune status, there is concern because echinacea has been shown to increase levels of tumor-necrosis-factor (TNF). This compound has been shown to stimulate replication of the HIV as well. At this time it appears wise for HIV-infected individuals to avoid echinacea until there is more research.

ALCOHOLISM

Alcoholism is defined by the World Health Organization as alcohol consumption by an individual that exceeds the limits accepted by the culture or injures health or social relationships. Current estimates indicate that alcoholism affects at least ten million people in the United States and causes 200,000 deaths each year, making alcoholism one of the most serious health problems today. The total number of people affected, either directly or indirectly, is much greater when you consider disruption of family life, automobile accidents (50 percent of fatal accidents involve a drinking driver), crime, decreased productivity, and mental and physical disease.

Dietary and Lifestyle Recommendations:

- Eliminate the consumption of alcohol, refined sugar, and coffee (both caffeinated and decaffeinated).
- Eat less saturated fat and cholesterol by reducing or eliminating the amounts of animal products in the diet.
- Increase the consumption of fiber-rich plant foods (fruits, vegetables, grains, legumes, and raw nuts and seeds).
- Do not smoke.
- Get regular exercise.
- Drink at least 48 ounces of water daily.

Primary Treatment Plan:

- Doctor's Choice (Male/Female) (Enzymatic Therapy)
  One tablet three times daily.
- Doctor's Choice Antioxidant Complex (Enzymatic Therapy)
  One to two tablets three times daily.
- Doctor's Choice Flax Oil Plus (Enzymatic Therapy) or Omega Twin (Barlean's)
  One tablespoon daily.
- Hypo-Ade (Enzymatic Therapy)
  One tablet three times daily.
- Stress-End (Enzymatic Therapy) or Ex-Stress (Nature's Way)
  One capsule three times daily.
- Liv-A-Tox (Enzymatic Therapy)
  One tablet three times daily.
- Super Milk Thistle (Enzymatic Therapy) or Thisilyn (Nature's Way)
  One or two capsules twice daily between meals.

Additional Recommendations:

- 1,000 mg of calcium and 500 mg of magnesium daily (any leading brand)
- L-glutamine (any leading brand)
  1,000 mg three times daily between meals.

Comments:

Alcohol consumption leads to hypoglycemia. The drop in blood sugar produces a craving for food, particularly foods which quickly elevate blood sugar, e.g., sugar and alcohol. Increased sugar consumption aggravates blood sugar control, particularly in the presence of alcohol. Hypoglycemia aggravates the mental and emotional problems of the alcoholic and the withdrawing alcoholic with such symptoms as sweating, tremor, rapid heartbeat, anxiety, hunger, dizziness, headache, visual disturbance, decreased mental function, confusion, and depression.

The herb silymarin and other lipotropic factors will help support liver function.

As with many serious conditions, prevention remains a key aspect. For more information on prevention, regarding addictions, refer to the side bar on the following page.

Healing Addictions:
Prevention is the best medicine of all!

"Addictions are illnesses with a strong social and behavioral component," according to *The Kellogg Report* by Joseph D. Beasley, M.D., and Jerry J. Swift, M.A. "While they are difficult to treat, they are preventable."

<u>Prevention</u>. As with many complicated illnesses, prevention seems to be the best medicine when it comes to healing addictions.

Obviously, regarding addictions, the best way to prevent becoming "hooked," is to avoid addictive behaviors and substances which can include:

• Prescription drugs such as Valium.
• "Street" drugs such as cocaine, heroin, etc.
• Alcohol.
• Caffeine and caffeine containing pills like diet pills.
• Sugar and sweets.
• Unhealthy relationships.
• Nicotine and marijuana.

It is also important to recognize if you have a genetic predisposition to becoming addicted. It has been shown that genetics are a key factor in determining a person's susceptibility to addictions. Realizing the genetic connection and taking special precautions to avoid addictive behavior is important.

Keeping the body healthy by eating a healthful diet and getting exercise will also help prevent addictions. Here are some dietary guidelines:

• Lots of fresh raw or lightly steamed vegetables.
• Unprocessed lean meats, chicken, fish, turkey; other proteins such as eggs, legumes, seeds, and nuts are also good.
• Whole-grain breads free of sugar and processed flour.
• Fresh fruits.
• Water—drink six to eight, eight-ounce glasses of bottled water daily.

Increasing physical activity and getting regular exercise is also a must. An effective exercise program should be consistent and last for a minimum of 20 minutes, three times a week.

By keeping the body healthy through diet and exercise, you will strengthen your body's immune and detoxification systems, allowing them to do their jobs effectively.

Given the damaging financial, physical, and emotional effects addictions have on our society, prevention has become even more critical. If you are worried about addictions, prevention should be your most important medicine.

ALZHEIMER'S DISEASE, SENILITY, and DEMENTIA

Senility and dementia refer to a general mental deterioration. In the elderly, this mental deterioration is often referred to as "senile dementia." Most often when this term is used, it describes a progressive deterioration of mental function, loss of short-term or recent memory, moodiness and irritability, self-centeredness, and childish behavior. Alzheimer's disease is the best known and most feared type of dementia. Alzheimer's disease can occur at any age, but most commonly after age 50. Symptoms occurring before age 65 are designated pre-senile dementia of the Alzheimer's type (PDAT). After age 65, it's senile dementia of the Alzheimer's type (SDAT). Current diagnosis of Alzheimer's disease is extremely difficult as the only definitive diagnosis is after-death biopsy of the brain.

Alzheimer's disease is characterized by the general destruction of nerve cells in several key areas of the brain devoted to mental functions. This results in neurofibrillary tangles and plaque formation. The disease's clinical features are believed to be related to a decrease in acetylcholine which functions as a transmitting agent in the brain, although there is a general reduction in the concentration of all neurotransmitting substances.

After death studies have demonstrated that about 50 percent of all cases of dementia are the result of Alzheimer's disease. This statistic means approximately 50 percent of dementia patients do not have Alzheimer's. It is not known to what degree patients are erroneously diagnosed as having Alzheimer's, or some other dementia, but it is estimated to be a significant number. Fortunately, the following treatment plan will provide benefit to those individuals with many forms of dementia.

Dietary and Lifestyle Recommendations:

• Avoid aluminum (found in many antiperspirants, antacids, and cookware).
• Follow a general healthful dietary and lifestyle plan.

Primary Treatment Plan:

• Doctor's Choice (Male/Female) (Enzymatic Therapy)
    One tablet three times daily.

- Doctor's Choice Antioxidant Complex (Enzymatic Therapy)
    One to two capsules three times daily.
- Doctor's Choice Flax Oil Plus (Enzymatic Therapy) or Omega Twin (Barlean's)
    One tablespoon daily.
- Ginkgo Phytosome (Enzymatic Therapy)
    One capsule three times daily.
- Phosphatidylserine (Enzymatic Therapy)
    One capsule three times daily.
- Active-B12 (Enzymatic Therapy)
    One tablet twice daily.

Additional Recommendations:

- A hair mineral analysis will rule out high lead, aluminum, or other metals.
- BIOMAG + Ginkgo (Lehning Laboratories—Homeopathic)
    One tablet twice daily.
- Keylex, a granular phophatidylcholine (Harmony)
    Three to five tablespoons daily.

Comments:

Virtually any nutrient deficiency can result in impaired mental function. Nutritional status has been shown to be the major factor determining mental function in people over the age of 60. Better nutritional status means better memory and mental function. Correcting an underlying nutritional deficiency can restore normal mental function. A particularly important nutrient in Alzheimer's disease patients is vitamin B12. Vitamin B12 works together with folic acid in the manufacture of several nerve transmitters as well as in nerve cell replication. B12 levels are significantly low, and vitamin B12 deficiency significantly common in patients with Alzheimer's disease. Patients with severe mental disorders as a result of a B12 deficiency have had complete recovery upon B12 supplementation. Methylcobalamin is the most active form of vitamin B12.

ANEMIA

Anemia refers to a condition in which the blood is deficient in red blood cells or the hemoglobin (iron containing) portion of red blood cells. The primary function of the red blood cell (RBC) is to transport oxygen from the lungs to the tissues of the body where they exchange the oxygen for carbon dioxide. The symptoms of anemia, such as extreme fatigue, reflect both a lack of oxygen being delivered to tissues and a build-up of carbon dioxide.

There are several different types of anemia. The major categories are:
—Anemias due to excessive blood loss.
—Anemias due to excessive red blood cell destruction.
—Anemias due to deficient red blood cell production.

The most common anemias fall into the category of deficient red blood cell production. In most cases, anemia is secondary to blood loss or a nutrient deficiency. Iron deficiency is, by far, the most common nutritional cause of anemia. Deficiencies of folic acid or vitamin B12 can also lead to anemia.

NOTE: Any case of anemia should be properly diagnosed by a physician to identify the cause. Treatment must be directed at the underlying cause.

Primary Treatment Plan:

Any Anemia Including Iron Deficiency Anemia:
• Ultimate Iron (Enzymatic Therapy)
    Two capsules twice daily.

Folic Acid Deficiency Anemia:
• Folic Acid (Carlson Labs)
    400 mcg of folic acid twice daily.

Vitamin B12 Deficiency Anemia:
• Active-B12 (Enzymatic Therapy)
    One tablet twice daily.

Additional Recommendations:

• Liquid Liver Extract (Enzymatic Therapy)
    One to three capsules daily before meals.

- Iron + Herbs, liquid formula (Flora)
    As directed.
- Liquid Iron (Natrol)
    As directed.

Comments:

Liquid Liver Extract or Ultimate Iron can be used with any type of anemia. Each capsule of Ultimate Iron contains 30 mg of ferrous succinate and 250 mg of liquid liver fractions. Ultimate Iron provides highly absorbable iron and is relatively free from the side effects (nausea, constipation or diarrhea, etc.) common to other iron supplements.

A key advantage to Ultimate Iron and Liquid Liver Extract is that they are rich in "heme" iron. There are two forms of dietary iron, "heme" iron and "non-heme" iron. "Heme" iron is the most efficiently absorbed form of iron. It is iron bound to hemoglobin and myoglobin. While heme iron is absorbed intact, non-heme iron is dependent upon ionization and complex transport mechanisms. A breakdown of these mechanisms can reduce your body's ability to uptake non-heme iron. In addition, non-heme iron is extremely susceptible to blocking agents such as fiber, phosphates, calcium, tannates, and preservatives. Heme iron is not affected by these factors.

In addition to iron, Ultimate Iron provides other blood-building nutrients: vitamin C, folic acid, vitamin B12, and fat-soluble chlorophyll. It is a very good formula for any type of anemia as it provides many factors necessary for the manufacture of red blood cells.

If liquid iron formulations are preferred, Iron + Herbs (Flora) or Liquid Iron (Natrol) is recommended.

ANGINA

Angina describes a squeezing or pressure-like pain in the chest. Angina is caused by an insufficient supply of oxygen to the heart muscle. Since physical exertion and stress cause an increased need for oxygen by the heart, symptoms of angina are often preceded by these factors. The pain may radiate to the left shoulder blade, left arm, or jaw. The pain typically lasts for anywhere from one to 20 minutes.

Angina is almost always due to the build-up of cholesterol-containing plaque which progressively narrows and ultimately blocks the blood vessels supplying the heart--the coronary arteries. This blockage results in a decreased blood and oxygen supply to the heart tissue. When the flow of oxygen to the heart muscle is substantially reduced, or when there is an increased need by the heart, it results in angina.

The same dosages for angina are also useful in arrhythmia (altered heart rate or rhythm).

Dietary and Lifestyle Recommendations:

- Eat less saturated fat and cholesterol by reducing or eliminating the amounts of animal products in the diet.
- Increase the consumption of fiber-rich plant foods (fruits, vegetables, grains, legumes, and raw nuts and seeds).
- Achieve ideal body weight.
- Regular aerobic exercise under medical supervision.
- Do not smoke.
- Eliminate the consumption of coffee (both caffeinated and decaffeinated).
- Practice relaxation techniques.

Primary Treatment Plan:

- Doctor's Choice (Male/Female) (Enzymatic Therapy)
     One tablet three times daily.
- Doctor's Choice Antioxidant Complex (Enzymatic Therapy)
     One to two capsules three times daily.
- Doctor's Choice Flax Oil Plus (Enzymatic Therapy) or Omega Twin (Barlean's)
     One tablespoon daily.
- Oral Nutrient Chelates (Enzymatic Therapy)
     Three tablets three times daily for one month or longer if the angina has not yet been relieved. Reduce to two tablets three times daily after one month if there are no symptoms. Maintain this dosage for an additional six months, then reduce to one tablet three times daily indefinitely.

(continued on page 22)

Heart disease:
Magnesium plays important role in heart health.

Myocardial infarction is caused by partial or complete obstruction of one or more of the coronary arteries. A recent study featured in *The Lancet* examined the effect of intravenous magnesium sulfate in acute myocardial infarction.

The study showed that after nearly three years of follow-up, heart disease was reduced by 21 percent and all-cause mortality by 16 percent. The researchers concluded that "magnesium has many functions that could benefit patients with acute myocardial infarction."

The report says magnesium regulates numerous important enzymes, including those involved with carbohydrate metabolism. In addition, "myocardial infarction is associated with a decreased extracellular magnesium concentration... normal or high concentrations of magnesium promote restoration of high-energy phosphates and factor recovery from stunning." It is also believed that magnesium provides benefit because it prevents an intracellular build-up of sodium and calcium.

Some questions remain regarding magnesium and heart disease. This study does not address the benefits of early magnesium usage, nor the optimum dosage of supplemental magnesium.

The researchers conclusively recommended, however, that specifically regarding myocardial infarction, all patients should receive intravenous magnesium within six hours of onset. "...we cannot wait for the laboratory report...there is no reason to go without other therapies, including magnesium..." concluded the researchers.
—*The Lancet,* Vol. 343, April 1994.

- Herbal H Complex (Enzymatic Therapy)

    Two capsules three times daily for one month or longer if the angina has not yet been relieved. Reduce to one capsule three times daily after one month if no symptoms of angina. After four months of use, switch to Hawthorn Phytosome (Enzymatic Therapy) at a dosage of one capsule three times daily.
- Garlinase 4000 (Enzymatic Therapy)

    one tablet daily.

Additional Recommendations:

- CoQ10 (Source Naturals)

    100 mg daily.
- L-Carnitine (Twin Laboratories)

    500 mg three times daily.
- Vitamin E (Carlson Labs)

    400 IU daily.

Comments:

Angina is a serious condition that requires strict medical supervision. In the severe case, as well as in the initial stages in the mild to moderate patient, prescription medications may be necessary. Eventually the condition should be able to be controlled with the help of natural measures. If there is significant blockage of the coronary artery, refer to the American College of Advancement in Medicine (ACAM), 23121 Verdugo Drive, Suite 204, Laguna Hills, CA, 92653, 1-800-532-3688 (outside California) or 1-800-435-6199 (inside California). Chelation therapy may also be an option. For more information or a list of physicians who perform chelation therapy contact the American Board of Chelation Therapy at 1-800-356-2228.

Magnesium supplementation has also been shown to improve heart function. Because magnesium must be combined with calcium in a proper ratio, a magnesium-calcium imbalance may increase the risk of heart disease. Supplemental magnesium may enable certain patients to decrease their dose of antiarrhythmic drugs; however, consult with a healthcare professional before making any changes.

Keep in mind, all garlic supplements are not created equal. For example, while you need only take one tablet of the Garlinase 4000, you would have to take nine tablets of the Kwai garlic product to achieve the same effect.

ANKYLOSING SPONDYLITIS
(follow recommendations for RHEUMATOID ARTHRITIS)

ANXIETY

Anxiety is defined as an unpleasant emotional state ranging from mild unease to intense fear. Anxiety differs from fear. Fear is a rational response to a real danger, while anxiety usually lacks a clear or realistic cause. Though some anxiety is normal and, in fact, healthy, higher levels of anxiety are not only uncomfortable, they can lead to significant problems.

Anxiety is often accompanied by a variety of symptoms. The most common symptoms relate to the chest. These include heart palpitations (awareness of a more forceful or fast heartbeat), throbbing or stabbing pains, a feeling of tightness and inability to take in enough air, and a tendency to sigh or hyperventilate. Anxiety can cause tension in the muscles of the back and neck and can lead to headaches, back pains, and muscle spasms. Other symptoms can include excessive sweating, dryness of mouth, dizziness, and symptoms of the irritable bowel syndrome.

Dietary and Lifestyle Recommendations:

- Eliminate the intake of caffeine, alcohol, and sugar.
- Identify and control food allergies.
- Perform a relaxation exercise (deep breathing, meditation, prayer, visualization, etc.) for 10 to 15 minutes each day.
- Get regular exercise.

Primary Treatment Plan:

- Doctor's Choice (Male/Female) (Enzymatic Therapy)
    One tablet three times daily.
- Doctor's Choice Flax Oil Plus (Enzymatic Therapy) or Omega Twin (Barlean's)
    One tablespoon daily.

- Stress-End (Enzymatic Therapy) or Ex-Stress (Nature's Way)
   One capsule three times daily.
- Anti-Anxiety (Lehning Labs—homeopathic)
   20 drops in two to three ounces of water three to four times per day.
- KavaTone (Enzymatic Therapy)
   One capsule three times daily.

Additional Recommendations:

- Gamma-aminobutyric acid (GABA), an amino acid, (any leading brand)
   750 to 1,000 mg daily
- Nervosan (Bioforce—homeopathic)
   As directed.
- Liquid Kalm (Natrol)
   As directed.

Comments:

Caffeine must be avoided by patients with anxiety or depression. Caffeine is a stimulant. Even small amounts of caffeine, as found in decaffeinated coffee, is enough to affect some people adversely and produce symptoms of anxiety or depression.

The above treatment plan also applies to panic attacks. If anxiety is accompanied by depression, refer to that section of this book.

ARTHRITIS

(see GOUT, OSTEOARTHRITIS, or RHEUMATOID ARTHRITIS)

ARRHYTHMIAS

(follow recommendations for ANGINA)

ASTHMA

Asthma is an allergic disorder characterized by spasm of the bronchial tubes and excessive excretion of a viscous mucous in the lungs. This can lead to difficult breathing. Asthma occurs as recurrent attacks which range from mild wheezing to a life-threatening inability to breathe.

The number of Americans suffering from asthma and other allergies has risen dramatically over the last 15 years. Some possible reasons include: increased stress on the immune system due to greater chemical pollution in the air, water, and food; earlier weaning and earlier introduction of solid foods to infants; food additives; and genetic manipulation of plants resulting in food components with greater allergenic tendencies.

Dietary and Lifestyle Recommendations:

- Eliminate food allergies.
- Avoid air-borne allergens.
- Follow a vegetarian diet.
- Drink at least 48 ounces of water daily.

Primary Treatment Plan:

- Doctor's Choice (Male/Female) (Enzymatic Therapy)
    One tablet three times daily.
- Doctor's Choice Antioxidant Complex (Enzymatic Therapy)
    One to two capsules three times daily.
- Doctor's Choice Flax Oil Plus (Enzymatic Therapy) or Omega Twin (Barlean's)
    One tablespoon daily.
- Vitamin C (any leading brand)
    10 to 30 mg for every 2 pounds body weight taken daily.
- Magnesium-Potassium Chelates (Enzymatic Therapy)
    One tablet three times daily.
- Air-Power (Enzymatic Therapy)
    Two tablets three times daily.
- As-Comp (Enzymatic Therapy) or Breathe-Aid (Nature's Way)
    As directed.
- Asthma and Allergy Formula (Lehning Labs—homeopathic)
    As directed.

Additional Recommendations:

- Adrenal-Cortex Complex (Enzymatic Therapy)
    One to three capsules daily.
- Vitamin B6 (any leading brand)
    50 mg two times daily.
- Active B-12 (Enzymatic Therapy)
    1 to 3 mg daily.
- Asthmasan (Bioforce—homeopathic)
    As directed.

Comments:

Food allergies are a major cause of asthma, especially in children. Milk, corn, wheat, citrus, peanuts, eggs, chocolate, food colorings, and food additives are the major culprits. In childhood asthma, eliminating food allergies and food additives is often all that is needed.

Air-borne allergens such as pollen, dander, and dust mites are often difficult to avoid entirely; however, measures can be taken to reduce exposure. Make the bedroom as allergy proof as possible. Encase the mattress in an allergen-proof plastic; wash sheets, blankets, pillow cases, and mattress pads every week; and consider using bedding material made from Ventflex, a special hypoallergenic synthetic material.

For information on air purifiers and other products designed for people with allergies, contact Allergy Control Products at 1-800-422-DUST or National Allergy Supply at 1-800-522-1448.

ATHEROSCLEROSIS

(see CHOLESTEROL)

ATTENTION DEFICIT DISORDER

Attention deficit disorder (ADD) is the term currently used to describe a condition that has had multiple labels in the past. Included are "hyperactivity" and "learning disability." This condition describes three separate disorders: attention deficit disorder without hyperactivity, attention deficit disorder with hyperactivity, and attention deficit disorder—residual type. Residual attention deficit disorder (individuals 18 years or older) is viewed primarily as a continuation of the process. Attention deficit disorder with hyperactivity is the most common. About three percent of all school-age children carry this diagnosis. Boys are more likely to be given this diagnosis than girls. In fact, ten boys will have it for every one girl.

The characteristics of this disorder, in order of their frequency, are: hyperactivity; perceptual motor impairment; emotional instability; general coordination deficit; disorders of attention (short attention span, distractibility, lack of perseverance, failure to finish things off, not listening, poor concentration); impulsiveness (action before thought, abrupt shifts in activity, poor organizing, jumping up in class); disorders of memory and thinking; specific learning disabilities; disorders of speech and hearing; and neurological signs and electroencephalograph (EEG) irregularities.

To help the child with ADD, parents must become acutely aware of the child's emotional and physical environment at school and home. Also, what and when the child eats will reveal important information.

Dietary and Lifestyle Recommendations:

- Eliminate food allergies and food additives (refer to Dr. William Crook's book *Help for the Hyperactive Child,* or any of the excellent books on attention deficit disorder and hyperactivity written by Dr. Doris Rapp). Also, Meridian Valley Clinical Laboratory (1-206-859-8700) offers food allergy tests that measure both IgE and IgG antibodies for over 100 different foods, and comes with detailed dietary instructions, for a total cost of about $120.
- Reduce sugar and caffeine intake.
- Read labels and avoid foods with artificial colorings, flavorings, or chemical additives.

(continued on page 30)

The Ritalin Rage:
How is this drug affecting our children?

Dr. Smith (Lendon Smith, M.D., world-renowned retired physician and author from Portland, OR), Dr. Feingold (the late Ben F. Feingold, M.D., pioneer of the concept that eating artificial colorings, flavorings, and chemical additives cause ADD), and many other healthcare professionals believe the behavior of the child with attention deficit disorder (ADD) can be controlled without drug therapy. Unfortunately, far too many physicians, psychiatrists, teachers, and parents believe the drug Ritalin is the answer to many behavioral problems, including ADD.

During a 1994 newscast regarding a shortage of Ritalin, it was reported that Ritalin sales have increased more than 33 percent over the past year alone. An estimated 4 million children receive Ritalin in the United States today.

Ritalin is an amphetamine that works to slow down children with ADD. *Prevention's New Encyclopedia of Common Diseases* states that "Amphetamines (such as Ritalin) only appear to calm the hyperactive child. What they really do is turn him/her into a robot."

According to the 1992 *Physician's Desk Reference* (PDR), here are just a few of the side effects of Ritalin:
- nervousness and insomnia
- anorexia and nausea
- blood pressure fluctuations
- dizziness
- headache
- drowsiness
- abdominal pain
- dermatitis and other skin rashes

The PDR warns that Ritalin should not be given to children under age six because "safety and efficacy in this age group have not been established." The PDR goes on to caution, "Sufficient data on safety and efficacy of long-term use of Ritalin in children are not yet available."

Because of these side effects and adverse reactions, Dr. Smith believes Ritalin should be a last resort, only used after all other options have been exhausted.

Unfortunately, many physicians believe Ritalin is their only option and are quick to prescribe it once a diagnosis has been made. "That's what I used to do," admitted Dr. Smith. After much research and just plain perception, Dr. Smith has found that ADD can be treated without Ritalin— or any drugs.

"The nutritional approach may be slower, but is much safer," said Dr. Smith.

It was reported in the *Health and Nutrition Update* (Autumn 1991) that a parent's advocate group in Atlanta, GA, sued the American Psychiatric Association because it has approved the use of Ritalin for behavior that can be observed in most normal children at some time or another. The article reports that similar lawsuits have been filed throughout the United States.

Parents who turn to Ritalin also complain that their doctors do not discuss the number of harmful side effects associated with Ritalin use. One complaint filed against the British Columbia College of Physicians and Surgeons claimed the psychiatrist told them Ritalin was "as safe as a vitamin."

The British Columbia Chapter of the Citizen's Commission on Human Rights believes that Ritalin simply masks the real causes of ADD and is only being used because it is a "quick fix."

In his exposé entitled *Ritalin: A Psychiatric Assault On Our Children*, writer Darrell Evans reports that the problem lies with the psychiatrists' definition of ADD. Of the fourteen symptoms listed in the psychiatrists' *Diagnostic and Statistical Manual of Mental Disorders*, many of them can be applied to normal children:

- often fidgets with hands or feet or squirms in seat
- is easily distracted by extraneous stimuli
- has difficulty playing quietly
- often talks excessively
- often acts before thinking
- has difficulty sticking to a play activity
- needs a lot of supervision
- runs about and climbs on things excessively

Although some may argue that these characteristics can lead to behavioral problems, do they really warrant the use of a serious drug?

Evans reported that Dr. Wendy Roberts, Research Coordinator at Toronto's Research Hospital for Sick Children, believes misdiagnosing ADD is a huge problem.

Dr. Roberts said that a small pilot study of 11 children diagnosed with attention deficit problems revealed that six had true attention problems, while the other five had learning disabilities or were actually gifted.

Choosing the least toxic route first will provide our children with a better chance at true and lasting health.

Primary Treatment Plan:

- Children's high-potency multi-vitamin/mineral formula
  (Kindervital by Flora or Liquid Children's Multi-Vitamin by Natrol)
  As directed.
- BIOMAG + Ginkgo (Lehning Labs—homeopathic)
  One tablet in morning and evening.
- DMG-B15-Plus (Enzymatic Therapy)
  One capsule two or three times daily.

Additional Recommendations:

- Hair mineral analysis. Numerous studies have shown children with ADD often have high body stores of heavy metals. If heavy metals are elevated, follow the dosages given under HEAVY METAL TOXICITY.
- Vitamin C (Carlson Labs powdered)
  500 mg daily.
- Herbs such as chamomile or St. John's wort may also be calming.
- Stress-End (Enzymatic Therapy)
  One capsule daily.
- Uncle Val, for sleep problems (Herbs for Kids)
  As directed.
- Auntie Cham calming formula (Herbs for Kids)
  As directed.

Comments:

Nutrient deficiencies exist in a significant number of children with attention deficit disorder and learning disabilities. Fortunately, correcting any underlying nutritional deficiency will result in an almost immediate improvement in mental function. Even when there is no true nutrient deficiency, taking vitamins and minerals may help improve mental function in children.

When dealing with children, taking the least toxic route first is recommended. Fortunately, there are many safe, natural products on the market to assist you. You may need to try a few different combinations to find what will work the best for your child.

BLADDER INFECTIONS

Over 20 percent of women develop a bladder infection each year. If not treated early and well, the infection may become chronic and spread to the kidneys. The typical symptoms of a bladder infection can include: a burning pain during urination; increased urinary frequency; nighttime urination; a turbid, foul-smelling or dark urine; and lower abdominal pain.

Most bladder infections are caused by bacteria, however the diagnosis of bladder infection by culturing the urine for bacteria is imprecise since clinical symptoms and the presence of significant amounts of bacteria in the urine do not always correlate well. Only 60 percent of women with the typical symptoms of urinary tract infection actually have significant levels of bacteria in their urine.

Dietary and Lifestyle Recommendations: (Prevention)

- Drink plenty of water (three quarts or more per day).
- Try to urinate as soon as possible after sexual intercourse.

Primary Treatment Plan: (Acute Infection)

- Krebs Cycle Chelates (Enzymatic Therapy)
    Two tablets four times daily.
- CranExtra (Enzymatic Therapy) or CranActin (Soloray)
    Two capsules four times daily.

Additional Recommendations:

- Aqua Flow (Enzymatic Therapy)
    Two capsules four times daily.
- Cystosan (Bioforce—homeopathic)
    As directed.

Comments:

Although many physicians and women believe acidifying the urine is the best approach, several arguments can be made for alkalinizing the urine. First of all, it is often very difficult to acidify the urine. Many popular methods of attempting to acidify the urine, such as ascorbic acid supplementation and the drinking of cranberry juice, have very little effect on pH at commonly prescribed doses.

The best argument for alkalinizing the urine is that it appears to be more effective, especially in women without evidence of bacteria in their urine. The best method of alkalinizing the urine appears to be the use of a multimineral formula where the minerals are chelated members of the Krebs cycle, such as citrate, malate, fumarate, and succinate.

CranExtra provides concentrated extracts of two cranberry species. This common cranberry extract is standardized to contain five percent anthocyanidins and 30 percent organic acids, including quinic, malic, citric and hippuric acids. The upland cranberry extract (also known as uva ursi or bearberry) is standardized to contain 20 percent arbutin.

BLOOD CLOTS

(see THROMBOPHLEBITIS)

BOILS

A boil is an inflamed, pus-filled area of skin, usually due to a hair follicle (the tine pit from which a hair grows) becoming infected with the Staphylococcus auereus bacteria. A boil will usually start as a painful, red lump. As it swells, it fills with pus and becomes rounded, with a yellowish tip (head). Common sites include the back of the neck and moist areas such as the armpits and groin. A more severe and extensive form of a boil is a carbuncle.

Practical measures should be taken to prevent the spread of infection, such as cleaning the affected area, taking showers instead of baths, and washing the face and hands several times a day. Towels, linens, and clothing should be kept away from other family members, to avoid spread to others. Do not burst a boil. This may spread infection to deeper tissues. A hot compress applied every two hours will relieve discomfort and hasten drainage and healing. If the boil is especially large or painful, consult your physician for proper drainage.

Primary Treatment Plan:

- Doctor's Choice (Male/Female) (Enzymatic Therapy)
  One tablet three times daily.
- Doctor's Choice Antioxidant Complex (Enzymatic Therapy)
  One to two capsules three times daily.
- Doctor's Choice Flax Oil Plus (Enzymatic Therapy) or Omega Twin (Barlean's)
  One tablespoon daily.
- Akne-Zyme (Enzymatic Therapy)
  One capsule twice daily.
  (Note: Do not use Akne-Zyme during pregnancy or when abdominal pain, nausea or vomiting are present. Akne-Zyme may cause temporary gas.)
- Hydrastine (Enzymatic Therapy) or Golden Seal Root (Nature's Herbs)
  Two capsules three times daily between meals.

Additional Recommendations:

- Zinc (any leading brand)
  100 to 150 mg daily for one month.
- Caster oil topical packs (Home Health or Heritage)
  As directed.

Comments:

Apply a hot compress over the area every two hours followed by a topical application of pure tea tree oil (Thursday Plantation).

BONE SPURS

Bone spurs most often occur on the heel. A spur is composed of a weak calcium structure and often reflects an over-alkaline condition.

Dietary and Lifestyle Guidelines:

- Avoid antacids and mineral formulas which feature calcium carbonate.
- Minerals chelated to weak acids like the Krebs cycle intermediates should be used.

- Drink at least 48 ounces of water daily.

Primary Treatment Plan:

- Acid-A-Cal (Enzymatic Therapy)
    Two capsules with each meal and at bedtime.

BRONCHITIS AND PNEUMONIA

Bronchitis refers to an infection or irritation of the bronchial tree, while pneumonia refers to infection or irritation of the lungs. Both are characterized by chills, fever, and chest pain. Pneumonia will show more signs of lung involvement (shallow breathing, cough, abnormal breath sounds, etc.). X-rays of patients with pneumonia will show infiltration of fluid and lymph in the lungs. Of the two conditions, pneumonia is by far the more serious. If you suspect you have pneumonia, see your doctor or visit your local emergency room for care.

Dietary and Lifestyle Guidelines:

- Avoid cigarette smoke and other respiratory irritants.
- Drink at least 48 ounces of water daily and get plenty of rest.
- Avoid sugar and dairy products.

Primary Treatment Plan: (Acute Treatment)

- ThymuPlex (Enzymatic Therapy)
    Two tablets twice daily.
- Vitamin C (any leading brand)
    500 to 1,000 mg every waking hour or to bowel tolerance.
- Hydrastine (Enzymatic Therapy) or Golden Seal Root (Nature's Herbs)
    Four capsules three times daily.
- Air-Power (Enzymatic Therapy) or Breathe Aid (Nature's Way)
    As directed.
- Bronchitis Formula (Lehning Labs—homeopathic)
    20 drops in 3 ounces of water every two to three hours, three to five times per day.

Additional Recommendations:

- A non-homeopathic bronchitis formula is Bronc Ease (Nature's Herbs)
  As directed.

Comments:

One of our main treatment goals in bronchitis and pneumonia is to help the lungs and air passages get rid of the excessive mucus. The following should be performed twice daily: Apply a heating pad, hot water bottle, or a mustard poultice to the chest for up to twenty minutes. A mustard poultice is made by mixing one part dry mustard with three parts flour and adding enough water to make a paste. The paste is then spread on thin cotton (an old pillow case works well) or cheesecloth, folded, and then placed on the chest. Check often as the mustard can cause blisters if left on too long. After application of the hot pack, perform postural drainage by lying with the top half of the body off the bed using the forearms as support. The position should be assumed for a five to 15 minute period while trying to cough and expectorate into a basin or newspaper on the floor.

BRUISES

Bruises are often a result of trauma. If bruises occur with only minor trauma, it usually reflects thinning of the dermis (the support structure just below the surface of the skin). Regardless of the cause of the bruising, the following recommendations can be of value.

Dietary and Lifestyle Recommendations:

- Consume a diet rich in flavonoids by increasing the intake of fresh berries, onions, and citrus fruit.
- Drink at least 48 ounces of water daily.

Primary Treatment Plan:

- Doctor's Choice (Male/Female) (Enzymatic Therapy)
  One tablet three times daily.

- Doctor's Choice Antioxidant Complex (Enzymatic Therapy)
    One to two capsules three times daily.
- Arnica Montana 1X homeopathic ointment (Hylands)
    Apply to area freely as needed a minimum of three to four times daily.
- Vitamin C (any leading brand)
    1,000 to 3,000 mg daily in divided dosages.
- Bromelain Plus (Enzymatic Therapy)
    One tablet twice daily between meals.

Additional Recommendations:

- Grape Seed (PCO) Phytosome (Enzymatic Therapy)
    As directed.
- Doctor's Choice Flax Oil Plus (Enzymatic Therapy) or Omega Twin (Barlean's)
    One tablespoon daily.
- Cellu-Var (Enzymatic Therapy)
    Two capsules twice daily.
- Cellu-Var Cream (Enzymatic Therapy)
    Apply to area twice daily.
- Tea Tree Oil (Thursday Plantation)
    As directed.

Comments:

Cellu-Var capsules contain three active components which have been shown to be clinically effective in reducing capillary fragility and the healing of bruises. Cellu-Var Cream contains escin, a compound from horse chestnut, which has been shown to be extremely useful in the healing of bruises. From a homeopathic perspective, Arnica Montana, is also very helpful in clearing up bruises. It is available in ointment or capsule form.

BURSITIS and TENDONITIS

Bursitis is inflammation of the bursa, the sac-like membrane which contains fluid which lubricates the joints. Bursitis may be secondary to trauma, strain, infection or arthritic conditions. The most common locations are shoulder, elbow, hip, buttocks, and lower knee. Occasionally the bursa can develop calcified deposits and become a chronic problem.

Tendonitis is an inflammatory condition of a tendon, usually resulting from a strain. Although acute tendonitis usually heals within a few days to two weeks, it may become chronic, in which case calcium salts will typically deposit along the tendon fibers. The tendons most commonly affected are the achilles (back of ankle), the biceps (front of shoulder), the pollicis brevis and longus (thumb), the upper patella (knee), the posterior tibial (inside of foot), and the rotator cuff (shoulder).

The most common cause of these conditions is sudden excessive tension on a tendon or bursa, although repeated trauma, such as from intense sports, can result in similar injury. Some tendonitis may have an anatomical basis, in that the grooves in which the tendons move may develop bone spurs or other mechanical abnormalities. Proper stretching and warm-up before exercise is recommended as an important preventive method.

Primary Treatment Plan:

- Curazyme (Enzymatic Therapy)
  Two to four capsules three times daily between meals.
- Myo-Tone (Enzymatic Therapy)
  One to two capsules three times daily with meals.
- Gingerall (Enzymatic Therapy)
  One to three capsules three times daily with meals.

Additional Recommendations:

- After an injury or sprain, immediate first-aid is very important. The acronym RICE summarizes the approach: Rest the injured part as soon as it is hurt to avoid further injury, Ice the area of pain to decrease swelling and bleeding, Compress the area with an elastic bandage to also limit swelling and bleeding, and Elevate the injured area above the level of the heart to increase drainage of fluids out of the injured area. Proper application of these procedures is important for optimal results. When icing, first cover the injury with a towel, then place an ice pack on it. Do not to wrap the injured part so tightly that circulation is impaired. The ice and compress should be applied for thirty minutes, followed by fifteen minutes without application to allow recirculation. Of course, for any serious injury, a physician should be consulted immediately. Indications for a physician include: severe pain, injuries to the joints, loss of function, and pain which persists for more than two weeks.

CANCER

Cancer is a very complex condition characterized by an unrestrained growth of cells. Most malignant cancers develop in organs, such as the lungs, breasts, prostate, pancreas, colon, etc., but they may also develop in other tissues and spread. Standard medical treatment of malignancies can include surgery, chemotherapy, and radiation. Chemotherapy and radiation expose healthy cells, as well as cancer cells, to free radical damage. The result is a great stress to antioxidant mechanisms and depletion of valuable antioxidant enzymes and nutrients. Therefore, nutritional support is vital as it provides additional antioxidants and accessory nutrients which can protect against the damaging effects of chemotherapy and radiation.

Keep in mind, many of the recommendations in this section can also apply to those interested in preventing cancer. Individuals with a family history or predisposition toward cancer should consider many of the following recommendations. In addition to a healthful diet and regular exercise, taking a high-quality antioxidant formula is especially important.

Dietary and Lifestyle Recommendations:

• Consume a high-fiber, plant-based diet.
• Consume 16 to 24 ounces of fresh vegetable juice daily.
• Get regular exercise.
• Watch comedies, read comics, and try to laugh often.
• Perform mind/body techniques (visualization, meditation, relaxation, etc.)

(continued on page 40)

Comprehensive Cancer Treatment:
The mind plays an important role in recovery.

Researchers have now discovered that the mind, specifically how we feel, act, and think, can play an important role in disease prevention and treatment. In 1989, *The Lancet* featured information exploring the effects of psychological intervention in the treatment of late-stage breast cancer. The results were fascinating.

For one year, 50 late-stage breast cancer patients were placed in a professionally led support group that met for 90 minutes once a week. Statistically, all of these patients should have died. At the end of the study, the average length of survival among the 50 women was twice as long as the 36 matched breast cancer patients who did not have the psychological support. All 36 of those women died, while even ten years later, three of the 50 women in the psychological support group were still alive.

It is interesting to note that this study was originally done to prove that the mind does not affect the body; however, researchers were surprised to learn that just the opposite was true.

In addition, the way we choose to respond to our health condition also affects our health outcomes. According to English researcher, Steven Greer, the attitude people have regarding their cancer determines the outcome more than any other single factor, including initial stage.

In Greer's 15-year study, patients with a fighting attitude had the best chance of survival. Interestingly, those in denial also did well. Stoic acceptance (indifference toward the disease) also did well. People with a helpless/hopeless attitude had the worse chance of survival. The attitudes of stoicism and helpless/hopelessness were not associated with a more advanced state or worse medical prognosis. In other words, there is reason to believe that the attitude affected the outcome rather than that the expected outcome affected the attitude.

At the end of the 15 years, it was shown that the survival rate of patients who chose to fight or deny was more than two and one-half times greater than the others.

If you are interested in incorporating mind/body techniques in your cancer treatment plan, you can refer to the book, *Getting Well Again* by O. Carl Simonton, M.D., and Stephanie Mathews-Simonton. The book includes information on guided imagery, relaxation, overcoming resentment, and goal setting. Other books, tapes, and videos along this same line are also available in health food stores and book stores throughout the United States.

Primary Treatment Plan:

- Doctor's Choice (Male/Female) (Enzymatic Therapy)
  One tablet three times daily.
- Doctor's Choice Antioxidant Complex (Enzymatic Therapy)
  One to two capsules three times daily.
- Doctor's Choice Flax Oil Plus (Enzymatic Therapy) or Omega Twin (Barlean's)
  One to two tablespoons daily.
- Carotene Complex (Enzymatic Therapy)
  Two to four capsules daily.
- ThymuPlex (Enzymatic Therapy)
  One or two tablets twice daily.
- Vitamin C (any leading brand)
  3,000 to 12,000 mg daily in divided dosages.
- Herbal Complex with Vitamin C (Enzymatic Therapy)
  Ten drops three times daily gradually increasing over a two month
  period to up to 30 drops six times daily.
- Super Milk Thistle (Enzymatic Therapy)
  Two capsules twice daily between meals. Continue for six months
  after the last chemotherapy or radiation treatment.
- CoQ10 (Source Naturals)
  100 to 300 mg daily during chemotherapy and continue for six
  months after the last chemotherapy treatment.

Additional Recommendations:

- Pau D'Arco Tea (Alta Health Products)
  Two to three times daily.
- For people having a difficult time eating or maintaining body weight,
  consider supplementing the diet with a high quality whey protein at the
  dosage recommendation of 1 gram protein per 2 pounds body weight.
- Flor-Essence (Flora) essiac herbal formula
  As directed.
- Cell-Guard antioxidant enzymes (Biotec)
  Consult your local health food store.
- Maitake D-Fraction (Nature's Answer)
  12 to 20 drops three times daily.

Comments:

There are many different forms of cancer. The dosages provided here are nonspecific, yet apply to most forms. These dosages are not intended to offer an alternative treatment for cancer. Instead, they are designed to augment other treatments whether conventional or alternative. Cancer is a very complex condition. The most successful cancer treatment plan is comprehensive, treating the mind, body, and spirit. Natural medicine can provide an important compliment to any cancer treatment plan. Consult with a natural healthcare physician for more information on how to naturally treat cancer. Many of the recommendations can also be used as prevention. For more information on cancer prevention, visit your local health food store.

Therapeutic (higher) dosages of specific supplements may be required for cancer patients as opposed to an individual who wants to prevent cancer. Get assistance from your local health food store or a natural healthcare provider to confirm dosages.

Genistein, the active compound in soy, has been shown to be an excellent cancer preventive, especially for breast, ovarian, and colon cancers. Soy is available in powdered drink mixes, tofu, soybeans, soy milk, and many other products. It is also available in capsule form. Gem-A-Steen by Carlson Labs contains genistein and daidzein, two soy isoflavones. Four capsules contain more than the total isoflavone content of 1/2 cup of tofu or one cup of soy milk.

CANDIDIASIS

Candida overgrowth is now becoming recognized as a complex medical syndrome known as the yeast syndrome or chronic candidiasis. This overgrowth is believed to cause a wide variety of symptoms in virtually every system of the body. The gastrointestinal, genitourinary, endocrine, nervous and immune systems are the most susceptible. Many illnesses can be traced to candida overgrowth.

To determine if candida overgrowth is contributing to your health problems, complete the questionnaire on the following pages.

(continued on page 46)

Candida Questionnaire:
Are your health concerns yeast-connected?

		Point Score
1.	Have you taken tetracyclines or other antibiotics for acne for 1 month (or longer)?	25
2.	Have you at any time in your life taken other broad spectrum antibiotics for respiratory, urinary, or other infections (for 2 months or longer, or in shorter courses four or more times in a 1-year period)?	20
3.	Have you taken a broad spectrum antibiotic drug, even a single course?	6
4.	Have you, at any time in your life, been bothered by persistent prostatitis, vaginitis, or other problems affecting your reproductive organs?	25
5.	Have you been pregnant:	
	2 or more times?	5
	1 time?	3
6.	Have you taken birth control pills:	
	For more than 2 years?	15
	For 6 months to 2 years?	8
7.	Have you taken prednisone or other cortisone-type drugs:	
	For more than 2 weeks?	15
	For 2 weeks or less?	6
8.	Does exposure to perfumes, insecticides, fabric shop odors and other chemicals provoke:	
	Moderate to severe symptoms?	20
	Mild symptoms?	5
9	Are your symptoms worse on damp, muggy days or in moldy places?	20
10.	Have you had athlete's foot, ring worm, other chronic fungal infections of the skin or nails? Have such infections been:	
	Severe or persistent?	20
	Mild to moderate?	10
11.	Do you crave sugar?	10
12.	Do you crave breads?	10
13.	Do you crave alcoholic beverages?	10
14.	Does tobacco smoke really bother you?	10

Total score section A

Section B: Major Symptoms

For each of your symptoms, enter the appropriate figure in the point score column:

If a symptom is occasional or mild   score 3 points
If a symptom is frequent and/or moderately severe   score 6 points
If a symptom is severe and/or disabling   score 9 points

Add total score and record it at the end of this section.

Point Score

1. Fatigue or lethargy
2. Feeling of being 'drained'
3. Poor memory
4. Feeling 'spacey' or unreal
5. Depression
6. Numbness, burning or tingling
7. Muscle aches
8. Muscle weakness or paralysis
9. Pain and/or swelling in joints
10. Abdominal pain
11. Constipation
12. Diarrhea
13. Bloating
14. Troublesome vaginal discharge
15. Persistent vaginal burning or itching
16. Prostatitis
17. Impotence
18. Loss of sexual desire
19. Endometriosis
20. Cramps and/or other menstrual irregularities
21. Premenstrual tension
22. Spots in front of eyes
23. Erratic vision

Total score, Section B

Candida Questionnaire Continued

Section C: Other symptoms

For each of your symptoms, enter the appropriate figure in the point score column:

If a symptom is occasional or mild   score 1 point
If a symptom is frequent and/or moderately severe   score 2 points
If a symptom is severe and/or disabling   score 3 points

Add total score and record it at the end of this section.

Point Score

1. Drowsiness
2. Irritability or jitteriness
3. Uncoordination
4. Inability to concentrate
5. Frequent mood swings
6. Headache
7. Dizziness/loss of balance
8. Pressure above ears, feeling of head swelling and tingling
9. Itching
10. Other rashes
11. Heartburn
12. Indigestion
13. Belching and intestinal gas
14. Mucus in stools
15. Hemorrhoids
16. Dry mouth
17. Rash or blisters in mouth
18. Bad breath
19. Joint swelling or arthritis
20. Nasal congestion or discharge
21. Postnasal drip
22. Nasal itching
23. Sore or dry mouth
24. Cough
25. Pain or tightness in chest
26. Wheezing or shortness of breath

27. Urgency or urinary frequency
28. Burning on urination
29. Failing vision
30. Burning or tearing of eyes
31. Recurrent infections or fluid in ears
32. Ear pain or deafness

       Total score, Section C

       Total score, Section A

       Total score, Section B

            Total Score

The total score will help you and your physician decide if your health problems are yeast-connected. Scores in women will run higher than men, as seven items in the questionnaire apply exclusively to women, while only two apply exclusively to men.

- Yeast-connected health problems are almost certainly present in women with scores over 180 and in men with scores over 140.
- Yeast-connected health problems are probably present in women with scores over 120 and in men with scores over 90.
- Yeast-connected health problems are possibly present in women with scores over 60 and in men with scores over 49.
- With scores of less than 60 in women and 40 in men, yeasts are less apt to cause health problems.

Note: For more information on candida, visit your local health food store or a natural medicine practitioner.

Source: *Encyclopedia of Natural Medicine* by Michael T. Murray, N.D., and Joseph Pizzorno, N.D.

Dietary and Lifestyle Recommendations:

- Eliminate the use of antibiotics, steroids, immune-suppressing drugs, and birth control pills (unless there is absolute medical necessity).
- Do not eat foods high in sugar.
- Do not eat foods with a high content of yeast or mold including alcoholic beverages, cheeses, dried fruits, melons and peanuts.
- Do not drink milk or eat milk products due to their high content of lactose (milk sugar) and trace levels of antibiotics.
- Avoid all known or suspected food allergies.

Primary Treatment Plan:

- Doctor's Choice (Male/Female) (Enzymatic Therapy)
  One tablet three times daily.
- Doctor's Choice Antioxidant Complex (Enzymatic Therapy)
  One to two capsules three times daily.
- Doctor's Choice Flax Oil Plus (Enzymatic Therapy) or Omega Twin (Barlean's)
  One to two tablespoons daily.
- ThymuPlex (Enzymatic Therapy)
  One or two tablets twice daily.
- Candida Formula (Enzymatic Therapy)
  One or two capsules twice daily between meals.
- Enzydophilus (Enzymatic Therapy)
  One capsule three times daily with meals for the first week.
  Thereafter, one capsule daily with a meal.
- Dietary Fiber (Enzymatic Therapy)
  Two to four capsules at night before going to bed.

Additional Recommendations:

- If a powdered fiber is preferred use Fiber Plus (Yerba Prima)
  One to two teaspoons in water or juice daily.

Comments:

Individuals with candidiasis often suffer from lack of hydrochloric acid or pancreatic enzymes. Please see the section on indigestion for further recommendations if the above protocol is not completely effective in eliminating gastrointestinal symptoms of candidiasis. A comprehensive candidiasis program should include dietary changes, detoxification, digestion support, and immune system support. For more information about candida, write to the Candida Research and Information Foundation, P.O. Box 2719, Castro Valley, CA 94546.

CANKER SORES

Canker sores are shallow, painful ulcers found anywhere in the mouth cavity. They can be single or clustered and are anywhere from 1 to 15 mm in diameter. The ulcers are surrounded by a reddened border, and are often covered by a white membrane. An occasional canker sore may be the result of trauma from your toothbrush. Such an ulcer will usually resolve itself in seven to 21 days. For many people, however, canker sores are recurrent. Canker sores are often confused with cold sores. However, cold sores most often occur on the border of the lips and are linked to the herpes virus.

Dietary and Lifestyle Recommendations:

- Eliminate wheat and dairy products from the diet as most individuals with recurrent canker sores are sensitive to these foods.
- Identify and eliminate food allergies.

Primary Treatment Plan:

- Doctor's Choice (Male/Female) (Enzymatic Therapy)
    One tablet three times daily.
- Oral Basics (Enzymatic Therapy)
    One or two tablets three times daily.
- DGL (Enzymatic Therapy)
    Two to four tablets twenty minutes before meals.
- Ionized Calcium with Magnesium (Enzymatic Therapy)
    Three capsules two or three times daily.

Additional Recommendation:

- Rinse mouth with Oral Basics Mouthwash (Enzymatic Therapy)
  Twice daily.

CARPAL TUNNEL SYNDROME

Carpal tunnel syndrome is a common painful disorder caused by compression of the median nerve as it passes between the bones and ligaments of the wrist. Compression of the nerve causes weakness, pain when gripping, and burning, tingling, or aching. The sensation may radiate to the forearm and shoulder. Symptoms may be occasional or constant. They usually occur most at night. Carpal tunnel syndrome is found most commonly in people who perform repetitive, strenuous work with their hands such as grocery store clerks and carpenters.

Primary Treatment Plan:

- Doctor's Choice (Male/Female) (Enzymatic Therapy)
  One tablet three times daily.
- Doctor's Choice Antioxidant Complex (Enzymatic Therapy)
  One to two capsules three times daily.
- Doctor's Choice Flax Oil Plus (Enzymatic Therapy) or Omega Twin (Barlean's)
  One to two tablespoons daily.
- Vitamin B6 (any leading brand)
  100 mg daily.

Additional Recommendations:

- Curazyme (Enzymatic Therapy)
  Two to four capsules two times daily.
- If Curazyme is not used, take Bromelain (any leading brand)
  1,200 to 2,000 mcg daily.

Comments:

Vitamin B6 deficiency is a common finding in carpal tunnel syndrome. In double-blind, placebo controlled clinical studies, John Ellis, M.D., and Karl Folkers, Ph.D., and their coworkers at the University of Texas have successfully treated hundreds of patients suffering from carpal tunnel syndrome with vitamin B6. It may take as long as three months to produce a benefit, but vitamin B6 is effective. During the time it may take for vitamin B6 to work, use Curazyme, a curcumin/bromelain combination formula, to help alleviate pain and inflammation.

CATARACTS

Many older Americans suffer with cataracts. A cataract describes a loss of transparency of the lens of the eye. The origin of cataract formation is free radical damage to some of the sulfur containing proteins in the lens. These delicate protein fibers form white spots when they are damaged in a similar manner to the way sulfur rich proteins of eggs are when they are fried or boiled. The damaged lens will not be able to transmit light effectively to the retina.

Dietary and Lifestyle Recommendations:

• Avoid direct sunlight by wearing UV-blocking sunglasses when outdoors.
• Consume a diet rich in fruits and vegetables.
• Drink at least 48 ounces of water daily.

Primary Treatment Plan:

• Doctor's Choice (Male/Female) (Enzymatic Therapy)
    One tablet three times daily.

• Doctor's Choice Antioxidant Complex (Enzymatic Therapy)
    One to two capsules three times daily.

• Doctor's Choice Flax Oil Plus (Enzymatic Therapy) or Omega Twin (Barlean's)
    One to two tablespoons daily.

• CataComp (Enzymatic Therapy)
    One or two capsules three times daily.

• Vitamin C (Any leading brand)
    1,000 mg one to three times daily.

Additional Recommendations:

- I-Tone (Enzymatic Therapy) or Occudyne (Allergy Research)
    As directed.
- Cell Guard (Source Naturals)
    As directed.

Comments:

In the early stages of cataract formation, by following the above recommendations, significant improvement or no further development should be expected.

CELLULITE

The term "cellulite" is used to describe a cosmetic defect that consumes and tortures millions of women. It is a disorder of the subcutaneous tissue the tissue just below the surface of the skin. The subcutaneous tissue contains fat cells which vary in size and number from individual to individual. As women age, the supportive structures of the subcutaneous tissue tends to become thinner and looser. This allows fat cells to migrate into this layer which leads to the pitting and bulging as well as the granular "buckshot" feel of cellulite.

Cellulite is often associated with feelings of tightness and heaviness in areas affected (particularly the legs). Tenderness of the skin is quite apparent when the skin is pinched, pressed upon, or vigorously massaged.

Dietary and Lifestyle Factors:

- Achieve and maintain ideal body weight.
- Consume a diet rich in plant foods. Particular foods to enjoy are high-flavonoid foods such as berries, cherries, and citrus.
- Drink at least 48 ounces of water daily.
- Massage the affected areas regularly with the hand or brush.

Primary Treatment Plan:

- Doctor's Choice (Male/Female) (Enzymatic Therapy)
    One tablet three times daily.
- Doctor's Choice Antioxidant Complex (Enzymatic Therapy)
    One to two capsules three times daily.
- Doctor's Choice Flax Oil Plus (Enzymatic Therapy) or Omega Twin (Barlean's)
    One to two tablespoons daily.
- Cellu-Var (Enzymatic Therapy)
    Two capsules twice daily.

Additional Recommendations:

- Apply Cellu-Var Cream (Enzymatic Therapy)
    Twice daily (morning and evening) to affected areas.
- VinoStasin time-released tablet or cream (Klinga Pharma)
    (Note: This product is available in Germany, but may not be available in the United States at the time of this printing.)

Comments:

Do not expect miraculous results. It usually takes two to three months before significant improvement is noticed.

CEREBROVASCULAR INSUFFICIENCY

Cerebrovascular insufficiency refers to a lack of blood flow to the brain. Cerebrovascular insufficiency is extremely common in the elderly as a result of atherosclerosis. The atherosclerotic plaque pinches off the flow of blood to the brain. The major symptoms of cerebral vascular insufficiency are impaired mental performance, short-term memory loss, dizziness, headaches, ringing in the ears, and depression. These symptoms are extremely common in the elderly and are often referred to as "symptoms of aging."

Dietary and Lifestyle Recommendations:

- Eat less saturated fat and cholesterol by reducing or eliminating the amounts of animal products in the diet.
- Increase the consumption of fiber-rich plant foods (fruits, vegetables, grains, legumes, and raw nuts and seeds).
- Achieve ideal body weight.
- Regular aerobic exercise.
- Do not smoke.
- Eliminate the consumption of coffee (caffeinated and decaffeinated).
- Drink at least 48 ounces of water daily.

Primary Treatment Plan:

- Doctor's Choice (Male/Female) (Enzymatic Therapy)
    One tablet three times daily.
- Doctor's Choice Antioxidant Complex (Enzymatic Therapy)
    One to two capsules three times daily.
- Doctor's Choice Flax Oil Plus (Enzymatic Therapy) or Omega Twin (Barlean's)
    One tablespoon daily.
- Oral Nutrient Chelates (Enzymatic Therapy)
    Three tablets three times daily for one month or longer if the angina has not yet been relieved. Reduce to two tablets three times daily after one month of no symptoms of angina. Maintain this dosage for an additional six months, then reduce to one tablet three times daily indefinitely.
- Ginkgo Phytosome (Enzymatic Therapy)
    One capsule three times daily.
- Aorta-Glycan (Enzymatic Therapy)
    One capsule twice daily.

Additional Recommendations:

- If cholesterol levels are elevated follow recommendations in the section on CHOLESTEROL.
- Vitamin E (Carlson Labs)
    400 to 800 IU daily.

Comments:

If blockage of blood flow to the brain is severe, see a qualified EDTA chelation specialist by contacting the American College of Advancement in Medicine (ACAM), 23121 Verdugo Drive, Suite 204, Laguna Hills, CA, 92653, 1-800-532-3688 (outside California) or 1-800-435-6199 (inside California). Chelation therapy uses an IV solution to clear blockages.

CHEMOTHERAPY

(see CANCER)

CHOLESTEROL (ELEVATED BLOOD LEVELS)

An elevated cholesterol level is associated with an increased risk of developing atherosclerosis (hardening of the arteries), the major cause of death in the United States and has reached epidemic proportions throughout all of the Western world. Heart disease accounts for 36 percent of all deaths in the United States and ranks as our number one killer; strokes, another complication of atherosclerosis, are the third most common cause of death. All together, atherosclerosis is responsible for at least 43 percent of all deaths in the United States. In light of the fact that atherosclerosis is largely a disease of diet and lifestyle, it appears that many of these deaths could be significantly delayed through a healthy diet and lifestyle.

Foremost in the prevention and treatment of heart disease is the reduction of blood cholesterol levels. The evidence overwhelmingly demonstrates that elevated cholesterol levels greatly increase the risk of death due to heart disease. It is currently recommended that the total blood cholesterol level be less than 200 mg/dl. In addition, it is recommended that the LDL-cholesterol be less than 130 mg/dl, the HDL-cholesterol be greater than 35 mg/dl, and triglyceride levels be less than 150 mg/dl.

Dietary and Lifestyle Recommendations:

- Eat less saturated fat and cholesterol by reducing or eliminating the amounts of animal products in the diet.
- Increase the consumption of fiber-rich plant foods (fruits, vegetables, grains, legumes, and raw nuts and seeds).
- Achieve ideal body weight.
- Regular aerobic exercise.
- Do not smoke.
- Eliminate the consumption of coffee (caffeinated and decaffeinated).
- Drink at least 48 ounces of water daily.

Primary Treatment Plan:

- Doctor's Choice (Male/Female) (Enzymatic Therapy)
    One tablet three times daily.
- Doctor's Choice Antioxidant Complex (Enzymatic Therapy)
    One to two capsules three times daily.
- Doctor's Choice Flax Oil Plus (Enzymatic Therapy) or Omega Twin (Barlean's)
    One tablespoon daily.
- Hexaniacin (Enzymatic Therapy)
    One capsule (500 mg) three times daily with meals for two weeks then increase dosage to two capsules (1,000 mg) three times daily with meals. **NOTE: For diabetics, use Cholestoril (Enzymatic Therapy), one tablet three times daily.**
- Garlinase 4000 (Enzymatic Therapy)
    One tablet daily.

Additional Recommendations:

- GugulPlus (Enzymatic Therapy) or Gugulipid (Nature's Herbs)
    As directed.
- Carnitine (any leading brand)
    900 mg daily.

Comments:

Typically, this program will produce reductions in total cholesterol of 50 to 75 mg/dl in patients with initial total cholesterol levels above 250 mg/dl within the first two months. In patients with initial cholesterol levels above 300 mg/dl, it may take four to six months before cholesterol levels begin to reach recommended levels. Once a patient's cholesterol level is reduced below 200 mg/dl, reduce the dosage of niacin to 500 mg three times daily for two months. If the cholesterol levels creep up above 200 mg/dl, then the dosage of niacin is raised to 1,000 mg three times daily. If the cholesterol level remains below 200 mg/dl, then the niacin is withdrawn completely and the cholesterol levels are rechecked in two months with niacin therapy re-instituted if levels have moved up over 200 mg/dl. Garlic and flaxseed oil supplementation can be continued indefinitely.

Gugulipid Extract (Enzymatic Therapy) or GugulPlus (Enzymatic Therapy) can be added to the above protocol if after four months the total cholesterol remains above 250 mg/dl. Gugulipid Extract is also suitable for the rare patient who cannot tolerate inositol hexaniacinate. The dosage is one tablet three times daily.

Cholestoril (pantethine) is recommended primarily to individuals with elevated triglycerides or diabetics. Cholestoril is preferred in diabetics over Hexaniacin. Although there is no data concerning the possible adverse effects of inositol hexaniacinate, niacin is known to adversely affect blood sugar control in some diabetics. Pantethine has demonstrated excellent effects in diabetics. It not only improves lipid parameters, but also normalizes platelet lipid composition, microviscosity, and function. The dosage is 300 mg three times daily.

CHRONIC FATIGUE SYNDROME

The chronic fatigue syndrome (CFS) is a newly-established syndrome that describes varying combinations of symptoms including recurrent sore throats, low grade fever, lymph node swelling, headache, muscle and joint pain, intestinal discomfort, emotional distress and/or depression, and loss of concentration.

Dietary and Lifestyle Recommendations:

- Identify and control food allergies.
- Eliminate consumption of sugar, caffeine, and alcohol.
- Breathe with the diaphragm and hold the body in a posture that is reflective of high energy.

- Drink at least 48 ounces of water daily.
- Follow a regular exercise program.

Primary Treatment Plan:

- Doctor's Choice (Male/Female) (Enzymatic Therapy)
    One tablet three times daily.
- Doctor's Choice Antioxidant Complex (Enzymatic Therapy)
    One to two capsules three times daily.
- Doctor's Choice Flax Oil Plus (Enzymatic Therapy) or Omega Twin (Barlean's)
    One tablespoon daily.
- Vitamin C E-mergen-C (Alacer)
    3,000 mg to 8,000 mg in divided doses each day.
- ThymuPlex (Enzymatic Therapy) or Thymulus (Enzymatic Therapy)
    Two tablets or two capsules twice daily.
- Raw Adrenal (Enzymatic Therapy)
    One capsule three times daily with meals.
- Liquid Liver Extract with Siberian Ginseng (Enzymatic Therapy)
    One to three capsules three times daily with meals.
- Anti-Fatigue (Lehning Laboratories—homeopathic)
    As directed.

Additional Recommendations:

- Consider St. John's Wort Extract (Enzymatic Therapy) if there is depression or poor sleep quality. One capsule three times daily.
- Vitamin E (Carlson Labs)
    1,200 IU daily.

Comments:

Chronic fatigue can be the result of many underlying factors. For more information, refer to Dr. Michael T. Murray's book, *Chronic Fatigue Syndrome* for a complete description of these factors (part of the *Getting Well Naturally Series* from Prima Publishing, 1994) in Appendix IV of this book.

COLD SORES

Cold sores are caused by the herpes virus. They are characterized by the appearance of single or multiple clusters of small blisters filled with a clear fluid on a reddened base. Cold sores differ from genital herpes in that the strain of virus is different. Cold sores are usually caused by Herpes simplex virus 1 (HSV1) while genital herpes is usually caused by the type 2 virus (HSV2). Most people, perhaps as high as 90 percent worldwide, are infected by HSV1. After the initial infection, the virus becomes dormant in the nerve cells in most people. In others, however, it can be reactivated. This causes recurring outbreaks usually following minor infections, trauma, stress, and sun exposure.

Dietary and Lifestyle Recommendations:

• Consume a diet which focuses on whole, unprocessed foods (whole grains, legumes, vegetables, and fruits).
• Avoid high arginine-containing foods (chocolate, peanuts, almonds, other nuts, and seeds).
• Eliminate the intake of alcohol, caffeine, and sugar.
• Identify and control food allergies.
• Drink at least 48 ounces of water daily.
• Get regular exercise.
• Perform a relaxation exercise (deep breathing, meditation, prayer, visualization, etc.) for 10 to 15 minutes each day.

Primary Treatment Plan:

• Doctor's Choice (Male/Female) (Enzymatic Therapy)
    One tablet three times daily.
• Doctor's Choice Antioxidant Complex (Enzymatic Therapy)
    One to two capsules three times daily.
• Doctor's Choice Flax Oil Plus (Enzymatic Therapy) or Omega Twin (Barlean's)
    One tablespoon daily.
• Vitamin C (any leading brand)
    3,000 mg to 8,000 mg in divided doses each day.
• ThymuPlex (Enzymatic Therapy)
    Two tablets twice daily.

Additional Recommendations:

- Apply Herpilyn (Enzymatic Therapy) to the lips two to four times a day during an active recurrence. Apply it fairly thick (1 to 2 mm). Detailed toxicology studies have demonstrated that it is extremely safe and suitable for long-term use. In fact, people with recurrent cold sores should use Herpilyn on a daily basis or as soon as the first tingling sensation of a cold sore is noticed.

COMMON COLD

The common cold is caused by a variety of viruses that infect the oral and nasal passages and the sinuses. The symptoms of a cold are well-known: fever, headaches, nasal congestion, sore throat or generalized malaise. Fortunately, there are many natural remedies that can help alleviate these symptoms.

Dietary and Lifestyle Recommendations:

- Rest.
- Drink plenty of liquids (focus on water, diluted vegetable juices, soups, and herb teas). Try to drink eight ounces of water every hour.
- Avoid sugar, including natural sugars such as honey, orange juice, and fructose, as simple sugars depress the immune system.

Primary Treatment Plan: (Acute Treatment)

- Vitamin C (any leading brand)
    500 to 1,000 mg every hour with a glass of water.
- EchinaFresh liquid (Enzymatic Therapy)
    Two to three droppersful three times daily.
- ThymuPlex (Enzymatic Therapy) or Vira-Plex (Enzymatic Therapy)
    Two tablets twice daily.
- Zinc lozenges (McZand Herbal)
    One every two hours.

Additional Recommendations:

- Cold & Flu Formula (Lehning Laboratories—homeopathic)
    As directed.
- Rhinitisan or Influaforce (Bioforce—homeopathic)
    As directed.
- For coughing, Biotussin (Bioforce—homeopathic)
    As directed.
- Also for coughing, Wild Cherry Supreme (Gaia Herbs, Inc.)
    As directed.

Comments:

Colds can be prevented by strengthening the immune system. Getting more than one or two colds a year or having a cold that lasts more than four to five days are signs of a weakened immune system. To strengthen the immune system, follow the supplement protocol given above, but reduce the dosage in half. Follow this treatment plan for eight weeks.

COLITIS

(see CROHN'S DISEASE and ULCERATIVE COLITIS)

CONSTIPATION

Constipation refers to difficulty in defecation. Constipation affects over four million people in the United States on a regular basis. The most common cause of constipation is a low-fiber diet.

Dietary and Lifestyle Recommendations:

- Increase the consumption of fiber-rich plant foods (fruits, vegetables, grains, legumes, and raw nuts and seeds).
- Drink six to eight glasses of water per day.

Primary Treatment Plan: (Acute Treatment)

- Daily Fiber (Enzymatic Therapy)
  Two to six capsules twice daily.
- Herbalax (Enzymatic Therapy)
  One to two capsules at bedtime.
- Green Magma (Green Foods)
  Two eight-ounce glasses daily.

Additional Recommendations:

- High doses of vitamin C are often an effective laxative.
- If you prefer a powdered fiber product use Fiber Plus (Yerba Prima)
  As directed.

Comments:

If you have been using stimulant laxatives, even natural ones like cascara or senna, you will need to "retrain" your bowels. Following are the recommended rules for reestablishing bowel regularity as presented in the *Encyclopedia of Natural Medicine* by Michael T. Murray, N.D. and Joseph Pizzorno, N.D. The recommended procedure will take four to six weeks.

Rules for Bowel Retraining

- Find and eliminate known causes of constipation.
- Never repress an urge to defecate.
- Eat a high-fiber diet, particularly fruits and vegetables.
- Drink six to eight glasses of fluid per day.
- Sit on the toilet at the same time every day (even when the urge to defecate is not present), preferably immediately after breakfast or exercise.
- Exercise at least twenty minutes, three times per week.
- Stop using laxatives (except as discussed below to reestablish bowel activity) and enemas.

Week one: Every night before bed take a stimulant laxative containing either cascara or senna. Take the lowest amount necessary to reliably ensure a bowel movement every morning.

| Weekly: | Each week decrease dosage by one-half. If constipation recurs, go back to the previous week's dosage. Decrease dosage if diarrhea occurs. |

CROHN'S DISEASE and ULCERATIVE COLITIS

Crohn's disease and ulcerative colitis are the two major categories of inflammatory bowel disease (IBD). Crohn's disease most often affects the ileum or terminal portion of the small intestine. Ulcerative colitis affects the lining of the colon. Both diseases are characterized by intestinal pain, diarrhea, and malabsorption of nutrients. Ulcerative colitis is slightly more common than Crohn's disease.

Dietary and Lifestyle Recommendations:

• Key recommendation = Identify and control food allergies.

Primary Treatment Plan:

• Doctor's Choice (Male/Female) (Enzymatic Therapy)
    One tablet three times daily.
• Doctor's Choice Antioxidant Complex (Enzymatic Therapy)
    One to two capsules three times daily.
• Doctor's Choice Flax Oil Plus (Enzymatic Therapy) or Omega Twin (Barlean's)
    One tablespoon daily.
• Vitamin C (any leading brand)
    3,000 mg to 8,000 mg in divided doses each day.
• Robert's Complex (Enzymatic Therapy)
    Two capsules three times daily with meals.
• Curazyme (Enzymatic Therapy)
    Two capsules three times daily before meals.
• Mega-Zyme (Enzymatic Therapy)
    Two to four capsules three times daily between meals.
• Green Magma (Green Foods)
    Two to three eight-ounce glasses daily.

Additional Recommendations:

- Take three to five grams of water-soluble fiber at bedtime.
- DGL (Enzymatic Therapy or Twin Labs)
  One to two chewable tablets 20 minutes before each meal.

Comments:

Diets which eliminate food allergies have proven to be extremely effective in the treatment of both Crohn's disease and ulcerative colitis. Meridian Valley Clinical Laboratory (1-206-859-8700) offers a food allergy test that measures both IgE and IgG antibodies for over 100 different foods along with detailed dietary instructions at a cost of about $120.

DEPRESSION

The official definition of "clinical" depression is based upon the following eight primary criteria:

1. Poor appetite with weight loss, or increased appetite with weight gain.
2. Insomnia or hypersomnia.
3. Physical hyperactivity or inactivity.
4. Loss of interest or pleasure in usual activities, or decrease in sex drive.
5. Loss of energy and feelings of fatigue.
6. Feelings of worthlessness, self-reproach or inappropriate guilt.
7. Diminished ability to think or concentrate.
8. Recurrent thoughts of death or suicide.

The presence of five of these eight symptoms definitely indicates depression. The individual with four is probably also depressed.

Dietary and Lifestyle Recommendations:

- Increase the consumption of fiber-rich plant foods (fruits, vegetables, grains, legumes, and raw nuts and seeds).
- Avoid the intake of caffeine, nicotine, other stimulants, and alcohol.
- Identify and control food allergies.

- Develop a positive, optimistic mental attitude by...
  —Setting goals
  —Using positive self-talk and affirmations
  —Asking yourself empowering questions
- Seek the help of a mental health professional.
- Exercise regularly.
- Perform a relaxation/stress reduction technique for 10 to 15 minutes daily.
- Find ways to interject humor and laughter in your life.

Primary Treatment Plan:

- Doctor's Choice (Male/Female) (Enzymatic Therapy)
  One tablet three times daily.
- Doctor's Choice Antioxidant Complex (Enzymatic Therapy)
  One to two capsules three times daily.
- Doctor's Choice Flax Oil Plus (Enzymatic Therapy) or Omega Twin (Barlean's)
  One tablespoon daily.
- St. John's Wort Extract (Enzymatic Therapy)
  One capsule three times daily.
- Folic acid (Carlson Labs)
  1,000 mcg daily.
- Active B-12 (Enzymatic Therapy)
  One to three mg daily.
- L-tyrosine (Carlson Labs)
  2,000 mg daily.

Additional Recommendations:

- If you are over age 50, Ginkgo Phytosome (Enzymatic Therapy), one capsule three times daily, is also recommended.
- For depression associated with menopause try Remifemin (Enzymatic Therapy) as directed.
- Phyto-Proz (Gaia Herbs, Inc.)
  As directed.

Comments:

St. John's wort extract (0.3 percent hypericin content) at a dosage of 300 mg three times daily has been shown to be as effective as standard antidepressant drugs (including Prozac) without side effects for mild to moderate depression. If you are currently on a prescription antidepressant drug, you must work with your doctor before discontinuing any drug. Discontinuing an antidepressant drug without medical supervision can be life-threatening. For more information refer to Dr. Michael T. Murray's book *Natural Alternatives to Prozac,* listed in Appendix IV of this book.

DERMATITIS

(see ECZEMA)

DETOXIFICATION

Toxic substances are in the air we breathe, the foods we eat, and the water we drink. It is believed that a person's health depends largely on his or her body's ability to efficiently eliminate these toxins from the system. This process is called the detoxification process. Fortunately, there are many ways to support the detoxification and elimination of harmful compounds. The importance of this process cannot be overstated. Many serious illnesses have been linked to pollutants and the body's inability to properly discard toxins.

Dietary and Lifestyle Recommendations:

- Fasting is one method used to detoxify the body. For more information on fasting refer to the *Encyclopedia of Natural Medicine* by Michael T. Murray, N.D., and Joseph Pizzorno, N.D. (Appendix IV).
- If you choose not to use the fasting method, your diet should be as natural as possible, high in fruits and vegetables and low in animal products.
- Drink at least two quarts of distilled or purified water daily.

Primary Treatment Plan:

- Doctor's Choice (Male/Female) (Enzymatic Therapy)
  As directed.

- Vitamin C (any leading brand)
    1,000 mg three times daily.
- Fiber Supplement (Enzymatic Therapy)
    1 to 2 tablespoons at night before retiring.
- Silymarin Phytosome (Enzymatic Therapy)
    As directed.

Additional Recommendations:

- Hydrastine (Enzymatic Therapy) or Golden Seal Root (Nature's Herbs)
    As directed.
- Sambu Cleanse (Flora) 3-day or 10-day program available
    As directed.
- Detox Program (BioForce)
    As directed.

DIABETES

According to The American Diabetes Association, although 13 million people in the United States have diabetes, less than one-half are even aware that they have the disease. Each year between 15,000 and 39,000 people lose their sight because of diabetes. In addition, people with diabetes are two to four times more likely to have heart disease and five times more likely to suffer a stroke. Diabetics also have a greatly increased risk of kidney disease and loss of nerve function. Diabetes mellitus is a metabolic disease characterized by an elevated level of blood sugar.

There are two major types of diabetes. Type I is often referred to as insulin dependent or juvenile-onset diabetes. Type II is also referred to as non-insulin dependent or adult-onset diabetes and is the less serious of the two types.

Differences Between Type I and Type II Diabetes

Features	Type I	Type II
Age at onset	Usually under 40	Usually over 40
Proportion of diabetics	Less than 10%	Greater than 90%
Seasonal trend	Fall and winter	None
Family history	Uncommon	Common
Appearance of symptoms	Rapid	Slow
Obesity at onset	Uncommon	Common
Insulin levels	Decreased	Usually elevated
Insulin resistance	Occasional	Often
Treatment with insulin	Always	Usually not required
Ketoacidosis	Frequent	Rare
Complications	Frequent	Frequent

There are other, less frequently encountered, types of diabetes. Secondary diabetes is a form of diabetes that is secondary to certain conditions and syndromes. These include pancreatic disease, hormone disturbances, drugs, and malnutrition. Gestational diabetes refers to glucose intolerance occurring during pregnancy.

Dietary and Lifestyle Recommendations:

- Consume a diet which focuses on whole, unprocessed foods (whole grains, legumes, vegetables, fruits, nuts, and seeds).
- Eliminate the intake of alcohol, caffeine, and sugar.
- Get regular exercise.

Primary Treatment Plan:

- Doctor's Choice (Male/Female) (Enzymatic Therapy)
    One tablet three times daily.
- Doctor's Choice Antioxidant Complex (Enzymatic Therapy)
    One to two tablets three times daily.
- Doctor's Choice Flax Oil Plus (Enzymatic Therapy) or Omega Twin (Barlean's)
    One tablespoon daily.

(continued on page 68)

The Sugar Blues:
Determine your status with this self-appraisal.

This brief questionnaire will help you determine whether you may be suffering from low blood sugar. Read over the symptoms to the right and mark them if they pertain to you with a 1 for mild symptoms, 2 for moderate symptoms that occur more frequently, and 3 for very severe symptoms that trouble you almost constantly.

A score of six from a combination of ones and two indicates the need for blood sugar support. A total of three or more threes is an indication that you should see your doctor.

With a score of 0 to 6 take one Hypo-Ade daily. Scores between 7 and 11 should take two tablets twice daily. And scores between 12 and 18 should take two tablets three times a day.

( ) Nervousness   ( ) Internal trembling

( ) Irritability   ( ) Palpitation of heart

( ) Exhaustion   ( ) Rapid pulse

( ) Faintness, dizziness   ( ) Antisocial

( ) Tremor, cold sweats   ( ) Indecisiveness

( ) Weak spells   ( ) Crying spells

( ) Depression   ( ) Lack of concentration

( ) Headache   ( ) Blurred vision

( ) Digestive disturbances ( ) Twitching, jerking of muscles

( ) Forgetfulness   ( ) Sighing and yawning

( ) Insomnia   ( ) Craves sweets

( ) Constant worrying   ( ) Nightmares

( ) Unprovoked anxiety   ( ) Phobias, fears

( ) Mental confusion   ( ) Suicidal intent

( ) Nervous breakdown   ( ) Convulsions

TOTAL _____

- Magnesium-Potassium Chelates (Enzymatic Therapy)
    One tablet two to three times daily with meals.
- Dia-Comp (Enzymatic Therapy)
    Two capsules three times daily with meals.
- Garlinase 4000 (Enzymatic Therapy)
    One tablet daily.

Additional Recommendations:

- If cholesterol or triglyceride levels are elevated, use Cholestoril (Enzymatic Therapy), one tablet three times daily.
- Vitamin E (Carlson Labs)
    400 to 600 IU daily.
- L-Glutamine (Solaray)
    As directed.

Comments:

The diabetic individual must be monitored carefully, particularly if he/she is on insulin or has relatively uncontrolled diabetes. Careful attention to symptoms, home glucose monitoring, and other blood tests are essential in monitoring the progress of the diabetic individual. It is important to recognize that as the diabetic individual employs some of the suggestions given above, drug dosages will have to be altered. The diabetic must establish a good working relationship with their doctor.

EAR INFECTIONS
and CHRONIC OTITIS MEDIA

An acute middle ear infection (acute otitis media) is characterized by a sharp, stabbing, dull, and/or throbbing pain in the ear. The pain is due to inflammation, swelling or infection of the middle ear. Acute ear infections are usually preceded by an upper respiratory infection or allergy. The organisms most commonly cultured from middle ear fluid during acute otitis media include *Streptococcus pneumoniae* (40 percent) and *Haemophilus influenzae* (25 percent).

Chronic otitis media (also known as serous, secretory or nonsuppurative otitis media with effusion, and "glue ear") refers to a constant swelling of the middle ear. Chronic otitis media affects 20 to 40 percent of children under the age of six. They account for over 50 percent of all visits to pediatricians.

Abnormal Eustachian tube function is the underlying cause in virtually all cases of otitis media. The Eustachian tube regulates gas pressure in the middle ear. It also protects the middle ear from nose and throat secretions and bacteria, and clears fluids from the middle ear. Swallowing causes active opening of the Eustachian tube due to the action of the surrounding muscles. Because this tube is smaller in diameter and more horizontal in infants and small children, they are particularly susceptible to Eustachian tube problems.

Obstruction of the Eustachian tube leads first to build-up from fluid in the blood, or serous build-up. If bacteria start to grow, this leads to bacterial infection. Obstruction results from a variety of causes. The tube can collapse due to weak tissues holding the tube in place and/or an abnormal opening mechanism. Or the collapse can occur due to allergic blockage with mucous, or infection.

Dietary and Lifestyle Recommendations:

• Avoid exposing child to cigarette smoke.
• Identify and eliminate food allergies. The most common allergens are milk, corn, wheat, citrus, eggs, chocolate and peanut butter.
• Strengthen the immune system by avoiding over-consumption of sugar.

Primary Treatment Plan: (Acute Phase)

• Vitamin C (any leading brand)
    10 mg for every pound of body weight every two hours. Crystalline vitamin C preparations work best. Hyland's offers vitamin C (25 mg) in a small chewable tablet for children.
• EchinaFresh (Enzymatic Therapy)
    One capsule three or four times daily.
    Note: capsules can be emptied into food in infants and young children.
• Enzydophilus (Enzymatic Therapy)
    One capsule daily. Note: capsule can be emptied into food in infants and young children.

- Children's high-potency multiple vitamin and mineral supplement
    (Kindervital by Floraor Liquid Children's Multi-Vitamin by Natrol)
    As directed.

Additional Recommendations:

- For acute ear infections in children, use a topical herbal-oil combination such as Ear Drops (Eclectic Institute). Apply a hot pack to the ear.
- Tea Tree Oil (Thursday Plantation) may also be used topically.

Comments:

Acute ear infections require medical supervision.

ECZEMA

Eczema, also known as atopic dermatitis, is an intensely itchy, inflammatory disease of the skin. It is commonly found on the face, wrists, and insides of the elbows and knees. Although it may occur at any age, it is most common in infants. It completely clears in half the cases by 18 months of age. Eczema affects 2.4 to 7 percent of the population and is often associated with asthma.

Dietary and Lifestyle Recommendations:

- Key recommendation = Identify and eliminate food allergies.
- Decrease consumption of animal foods with the exception of cold water fish (rich source of omega-3 fatty acids).

Primary Treatment Plan:

- Doctor's Choice (Male/Female) (Enzymatic Therapy)
    One tablet three times daily.
- Doctor's Choice Antioxidant Complex (Enzymatic Therapy)
    One to two tablets three times daily.
- Doctor's Choice Flax Oil Plus (Enzymatic Therapy) or Omega Twin (Barlean's)
    One tablespoon daily.

- Quercezyme-Plus (Enzymatic Therapy)
  One to two capsules five minutes before meals.
  Note: capsules can be emptied into food for infants and young children.
- Akne-Zyme (Enzymatic Therapy)
  One capsule twice daily with meals.

Additional Recommendations:

- Simicort (Enzymatic Therapy) or CamoCare (Abkit)
  Applied to the affected area two to three times daily.

Comments:

The causal role of food allergy in eczema is well established, especially in children. It has been concluded that perhaps 75 percent of cases of childhood eczema could be resolved merely by shifting some dietary factors. Cow's milk is a major culprit. Other key food allergens in eczema are eggs, tomatoes, and food preservatives and food colorings. Meridian Valley Clinical Laboratory (1-206-859-8700) offers food allergy tests that measure both IgE and IgG antibodies for over 100 different foods with detailed dietary instructions, at a cost of about $120.

ENDOMETRIOSIS

Endometriosis refers to a condition where fragments of the endometrium (the lining of the uterus) are found in other parts of the pelvic cavity. The symptoms of endometriosis can vary widely, with abnormal or heavy menstrual bleeding being the most common. Other possible symptoms include painful intercourse, symptoms of the irritable bowel syndrome (see IRRITABLE BOWEL SYNDROME), and rectal bleeding during the time of menses. Endometriosis is also a common cause of infertility.

Dietary and Lifestyle Recommendations:

- Consume a diet which focuses on whole, unprocessed foods (whole grains, legumes, vegetables, fruits, nuts, and seeds).
- A vegetarian diet may be helpful in reducing symptoms.

- Eliminate the intake of alcohol, caffeine, and sugar.
- Get regular exercise.

Primary Treatment Plan:

- Doctor's Choice for Women (Enzymatic Therapy)
    One tablet three times daily.
- Doctor's Choice Antioxidant Complex (Enzymatic Therapy)
    One to two tablets three times daily.
- Doctor's Choice Flax Oil Plus (Enzymatic Therapy) or Omega Twin (Barlean's)
    One tablespoon daily.
- Femtrol (Enzymatic Therapy)
    One or two capsules three times daily.

Additional Recommendations:

- If menstrual blood flow is quite heavy, add Liquid Liver Extract (Enzymatic Therapy) or Ultimate Iron (Enzymatic Therapy) to the supplement protocol.
- Silymarin (any leading brand) to improve liver function.
    As directed.

Comments:

If the endometriosis is severe, surgical removal of the material may be necessary. This may relieve symptoms and aid fertility. The connection between endometriosis and chronic candidiasis has been well documented. Refer to the section on candidiasis for further assistance.

FIBROID (Uterine)

A fibroid is a slow-growing benign tumor of the uterus that consists of smooth muscle bundles and connective tissue. Fibroids may vary in size from the size of a pea to that of a grapefruit. Fibroids occur in about 20 percent of women age 30 or older, making them the most common of tumors. The cause of fibroids is related to an abnormal response to estrogens.

Dietary and Lifestyle Recommendations:

- Consume a diet which focuses on whole, unprocessed foods (whole grains, legumes, vegetables, fruits, nuts, and seeds).
- Increase consumption of soy foods.
- Eliminate the intake of alcohol, caffeine, and sugar.
- Get regular exercise.
- Perform a relaxation exercise (deep breathing, meditation, prayer, visualization, etc.) for 10 to 15 minutes each day.
- Drink at least 48 ounces of water daily.

Primary Treatment Plan:

- Doctor's Choice for Women (Enzymatic Therapy)
  One tablet three times daily.
- Doctor's Choice Antioxidant Complex (Enzymatic Therapy)
  One to two capsules three times daily.
- Doctor's Choice Flax Oil Plus (Enzymatic Therapy) or Omega Twin (Barlean's)
  One to two tablespoons daily.
- Liv-A-Tox (Enzymatic Therapy)
  Two tablets three times daily with meals.
- Mega-Zyme (Enzymatic Therapy)
  Two to four tablets twice daily between meals.

Additional Recommendations:

- Remifemin (Enzymatic Therapy) specifically for women of menopausal age.
  Two tablets twice daily.

FIBROCYSTIC BREAST DISEASE

Fibrocystic breast disease (FBD), also known as cystic mastitis, is a mildly uncomfortable to severely painful benign cystic swelling of the breasts. Fibrocystic breast disease is very common. It affects 20 to 40 percent of premenopausal women. It is usually a component of the premenstrual syndrome (PMS) and is considered a minor risk factor for breast cancer. It is not as significant a factor as the classical breast cancer risk factors such as family history, early menarche, and late or no first pregnancy.

The development of fibrocystic breast disease is apparently due to an increased estrogen-to-progesterone ratio. With each menstrual cycle, there is a recurring hormonal stimulation of the breasts. As the hormone levels fall after a few days, the breasts normally return to their prestimulation size and function.

Dietary and Lifestyle Recommendations:

- Consume a diet which focuses on whole, unprocessed foods (whole grains, legumes, vegetables, fruits, nuts, and seeds).
- Increase consumption of soy foods.
- Eliminate the intake of coffee, tea, cola, chocolate, and caffeinated medications as well as alcohol and sugar.
- Drink at least 48 ounces of water daily.
- Get regular exercise.

Primary Treatment Plan:

- Doctor's Choice for Women (Enzymatic Therapy)
    One tablet three times daily.
- Doctor's Choice Antioxidant Complex (Enzymatic Therapy)
    One capsule three times daily.
- Doctor's Choice Flax Oil Plus (Enzymatic Therapy) or Omega Twin (Barlean's)
    One tablespoon daily.
- Female Balance (Enzymatic Therapy)
    One capsule three times daily.
- Mega-Zyme (Enzymatic Therapy)
    Two tablets three times daily between meals.
- Vitamin E (Carlson Labs)
    400 IU daily.

Additional Recommendations:

- Rule out hypothyroidism (see HYPOTHYROIDISM).

Comments:

Vitamin E has been shown to be effective in relieving fibrocystic breast disease in several clinical studies. There is now evidence that iodine may be beneficial in relieving pain associated with fibrocystic breast disease. For more information on this connection refer to the July 1995 issue of Drs. Jonathan Wright and Allan Gaby's newsletter, *Nutrition and Healing* (1-800-528-0559).

FOOD ALLERGY

Food allergies refer to an allergic reaction caused by the ingestion of a food. It is estimated by some experts that at least 60 percent of Americans suffer from negative reactions to food. Food allergies have been shown to be an important cause in a wide range of conditions.

<u>System</u>	<u>Symptoms and Diseases</u>
Gastrointestinal	Canker sores, celiac disease, chronic diarrhea, stomach ulcer, gas, gastritis, irritable colon, malabsorption, ulcerative colitis
Genitourinary	Bedwetting, bladder infections, kidney disease
Immune	Chronic infections, frequent ear infections
Brain	Anxiety, depression, hyperactivity, inability to concentrate, insomnia, irritability, mental confusion, personality change, seizures
Musculoskeletal	Bursitis, joint pain, low back pain
Respiratory	Asthma, chronic bronchitis, wheezing
Skin	Acne, eczema, hives, itching, skin rash
Miscellaneous	Irregular heartbeats, edema, fainting, fatigue, headache, hypoglycemia, itchy nose or throat, migraines, sinusitis

Dietary and Lifestyle Recommendations:

- An elimination diet can determine if food allergy is playing a major role in a particular health condition. The standard elimination diet consists of lamb, chicken, rice, banana, apple and a vegetable from the cabbage family. This diet is also called an oligoantigenic diet. The next step is the reintroduction of foods. A daily record book is necessary to keep a detailed journal of the dates when new foods are introduced, and any adverse responses in your body. Every second day a food can be reintroduced to the diet. If the food is one to which an individual is sensitive, the symptoms of the adverse response will reappear (often more strongly than before). The two-day wait before reintroducing the next food allows a period of up to 48 hours where such symptoms will likely be an adverse response to the reintroduced food.

Primary Treatment Plan:

- Doctor's Choice Flax Oil Plus (Enzymatic Therapy) or Omega Twin (Barlean's)
  One tablespoon daily.
- Quercezyme-Plus (Enzymatic Therapy)
  Two capsules five minutes before meals.
- Mega-Zyme (Enzymatic Therapy)
  Two to four tablets after each meal.

Additional Recommendations:

- If a person has multiple food allergies, follow the dosages given for INDIGESTION.
- Allergy Remedy (Lehning Laboratories—homeopathic)
  As directed.

Comments:

Meridian Valley Clinical Laboratory (1-206-859-8700) offers a food allergy test that measures both IgE and IgG antibodies, tests for over 100 different foods, comes with detailed dietary instructions and is reasonably priced at about $120.

GALLSTONES

Gallstones are an extremely common occurrence in the United States. Each year at least one million more Americans will develop gallstones and another 300,000 gallbladders will be removed. The critical factor in gallstone formation is the solubility of the bile within the gallbladder. Bile solubility is based on the relative concentrations of cholesterol, bile acids, phosphatidylcholine (lecithin) and water.

Dietary and Lifestyle Recommendations:

- Consume a diet which focuses on whole, unprocessed foods (whole grains, legumes, vegetables, fruits, nuts, and seeds).
- Eliminate the intake of milk.
- Eliminate consumption of food allergens (milk, onions, eggs, and chocolate are the most common in patients with symptoms).
- Drink at least 48 ounces of water daily.
- Avoid use of antacids.
- Get regular exercise.

Primary Treatment Plan:

- Doctor's Choice (Male/Female) (Enzymatic Therapy)
    One tablet three times daily.
- Doctor's Choice Antioxidant Complex (Enzymatic Therapy)
    One to two tablets three times daily.
- Symplex F (Standard Process) to stimulate bile flow
    Two tablets three to four times daily.
- Super Milk Thistle (Enzymatic Therapy)
    Two capsules twice daily between meals.
- Liv-A-Tox (Enzymatic Therapy)
    One to two tablets three times daily.
- Daily Fiber (Enzymatic Therapy)
    Two to three capsules with meals three times daily.

Additional Recommendations:

- Doctor's Choice Flax Oil Plus (Enzymatic Therapy) or Omega Twin (Barlean's)
    One tablespoon daily.

- Peppermint Plus (Enzymatic Therapy)

   One or two capsules twice daily between meals.
- Heptasan (Bioforce—homeopathic)

   As directed.

Comments:

A formula containing menthol and related terpenes (menthone, pinene, borneol, cineol, and camphene) has demonstrated efficacy in several studies in dissolving gallstones. This nonsurgical approach to gallstone removal offers an effective alternative to surgery and has been shown to be safe even when consumed for prolonged periods of time (up to four years). Terpenes, like menthol, help dissolve gallstones by reducing bile cholesterol levels while increasing bile acid and lecithin levels in the gallbladder. As menthol was the major component of this formula, peppermint oil, especially if enteric-coated, may offer similar benefits.

GLAUCOMA

Glaucoma refers to increased pressure within the eye that results from an imbalance between the production and outflow of fluid in the eye. Obstruction of outflow is the main cause of this imbalance in acute glaucoma. A number of physiological abnormalities have been observed in glaucomatous eyes. Sometimes there are unusual tissues at the back of the eye through which the optic nerve fibers and blood vessels pass. Abnormalities have been seen in the connective tissue network the eye fluid must pass through to leave the eye. Blood vessels in the eye have also been observed to be problematic. These changes may result in elevated inner eye pressure. Alternatively, they may lead to progressive loss of peripheral vision.

Glaucoma can be acute or chronic. Chronic glaucoma is much more common. In the United States there are approximately two million people with glaucoma, 25 percent of which is undetected. Ten percent have the acute closed-angle type and 90 percent is of the chronic open-angle type. In chronic glaucoma, there will not usually be any symptoms until there are significant elevations in pressure readings. Once the pressure of fluids in the eye reaches high enough levels, the person will experience a gradual loss of peripheral vision. In other words, the person will experience "tunnel vision." Extreme pain, blurring of vision, and severely reddened eyes may also be associated with this acute phase of the chronic condition.

Acute closed-angle glaucoma is a very serious condition. It is a medical emergency. Usually a person will experience severe throbbing pain in the eye. Vision will markedly blur. Nausea and vomiting are often also associated with its onset. A person who suspects this condition should go immediately to an ophthalmologist or hospital emergency room. Effective therapy must be started within 12 to 48 hours or permanent loss of vision will occur within three to five days.

Dietary and Lifestyle Recommendations:

- Consume a diet which focuses on whole, unprocessed foods (whole grains, legumes, vegetables, fruits, nuts, and seeds).
- Identify and eliminate consumption of food allergies (milk, onions, eggs, and chocolate are the most common in patients with symptoms).
- Drink at least 48 ounces of water daily.

Primary Treatment Plan:

- Doctor's Choice (Male/Female) (Enzymatic Therapy)
    One tablet three times daily.
- Doctor's Choice Antioxidant Complex (Enzymatic Therapy)
    One to two tablets three times daily.
- Doctor's Choice Flax Oil Plus (Enzymatic Therapy) or Omega Twin (Barlean's)
    One tablespoon daily.
- Vitamin C (any leading brand)
    500 mg for every 2.2 pounds of body weight in divided dosages (work up to this high dosage gradually).
- Herbal Flavonoids or Bilberry Extract (both by Enzymatic Therapy)
    One or two capsules three times daily.

Additional Recommendations:

- An alternative bilberry formula is Bilberry Complex (Bioforce)
    As directed.

Comments:

High doses of vitamin C have been shown to lower pressure levels on the inner eye in many clinical studies. Almost normal tension levels have been achieved in some patients who were unresponsive to standard drug therapies (acetazolamide and pilocarpine).

GOUT

Gout is a common type of arthritis caused by an increased concentration of uric acid in biological fluids. Uric acid is the final breakdown product of purine metabolism. Purines are made in the body and are also ingested in foods. In gout, uric acid crystals are deposited in joints, tendons, kidneys, and other tissues, where they cause considerable inflammation and damage.

Dietary and Lifestyle Recommendations:

- Eliminate alcohol intake.
- Follow a low purine diet.
- Achieve ideal body weight.
- Eliminate sugar and restrict intake of simple sugars (honey, fructose, fruits, fruit juices, etc.).
- Consume a diet which focuses on whole, unprocessed foods (whole grains, legumes, vegetables, nuts, and seeds).
- Drink at least 48 ounces of water daily.

Primary Treatment Plan:

- Doctor's Choice (Male/Female) (Enzymatic Therapy)
      One tablet three times daily.
- Doctor's Choice Antioxidant Complex (Enzymatic Therapy)
      One to two tablets three times daily.
- Doctor's Choice Flax Oil Plus (Enzymatic Therapy) or Omega Twin (Barlean's)
      One tablespoon daily.

- Cherry Fruit Extract (Enzymatic Therapy)
    One to two tablets three times daily.

Comments:

Most cases of gout can be treated effectively with diet alone.

HAIR AND SKIN

Radiant skin and vibrant, lively hair have long been associated with good health. In the past decade, it has become common knowledge that how well we take care of ourselves is mirrored in the condition of our skin and hair. Nutrition is vitally important to the health of our skin and hair.

Dietary and Lifestyle Recommendations:

- Utilize proper hygiene practices to keep your hair and skin healthy.
- Eat a wholesome diet, reducing fat and sugar intake.

Primary Treatment Plan:

- Hair and Skin Nutrition (Enzymatic Therapy)
    As directed. Provides a combination of important nutrients for the hair and skin. Will help restore hair growth for women with thinning hair.
- Vitamin E (Carlson Labs)
    400 IU daily.
- Vitamin C (any leading brand)
    500 mg three times daily.
- Alta Sil-X Silica (Alta Health Products) or Silica Gel (Abkit)
    As directed.

Additional Recommendations:

- VegeSil (Flora)
    As directed.

Comments:

To take care of your hair and skin properly, try to use hygiene products that are free of artificial colors, dyes, additives, and fragrances. Your local health food store provides a wealth of knowledge and many quality products to choose from.

HAYFEVER

The underlying mechanisms responsible for hayfever are very similar to those which produce asthma. Follow the recommendations given for ASTHMA.

HEADACHE

(also see MIGRAINE)

The most common form of headache is referred to as the "tension headache." Tension headaches are usually caused by a tightening of the muscles of the face, neck or scalp causing nerves to be pinched. Stress, poor posture, and hypoglycemia can trigger a tension headache. A tension headache is differentiated from a migraine in that it usually is associated with a steady, constant pain that starts at the forehead or back of head and can spread pain over the entire head, while a migraine tends to be a throbbing pain, which pounds sharply in the head of the sufferer.

Dietary and Lifestyle Recommendations:

- Consume a diet which focuses on whole, unprocessed foods (whole grains, legumes, vegetables, fruits, nuts, and seeds).
- Eliminate the intake of alcohol, caffeine, and sugar.
- Identify and control food allergies.
- Get regular exercise.

- Perform a relaxation exercise (deep breathing, meditation, prayer, visualization, etc.) for 10 to 15 minutes each day.
- Drink at least 48 ounces of water daily.

Primary Recommendations: (acute treatment)

- Magnesium-Potassium Chelates (Enzymatic Therapy)
     Two tablets (up to three times daily).
- Willowcin (Enzymatic Therapy)
     Two to six capsules (up to three times daily).

Additional Recommendations:

- Chiropractic adjustments can be quite useful in chronic tension headaches.
- Feverfew (Nature's Herbs)
     As directed.

HEART DISEASE

(see CHOLESTEROL or ANGINA)

HEMORRHOIDS

Hemorrhoids are basically varicose veins of the rectum. They may be near the beginning of the anal canal (internal hemorrhoids) or at the anal opening (external hemorrhoids). Because the venous system supplying the rectal area contains no valves, factors which increase venous congestion in the region can precipitate hemorrhoid formation. This includes increasing intra-abdominal pressure (e.g., defecation, pregnancy, coughing, sneezing, vomiting, physical exertion, and portal hypertension due to cirrhosis), a low-fiber diet-induced increase in straining during defecation, and standing or sitting for prolonged periods of time.

The symptoms most often associated with hemorrhoids include itching, burning, pain, inflammation, irritation, swelling, bleeding, and seepage.

Dietary and Lifestyle Recommendations:

- Consume a diet which focuses on whole, unprocessed foods (whole grains, legumes, vegetables, fruits, nuts, and seeds).
- Get regular exercise.
- Drink at least 48 ounces of water daily.

Primary Treatment Plan:

- Daily Fiber (Enzymatic Therapy)
    Two capsules with meals three times daily.
- Cellu-Var (Enzymatic Therapy)
    Two capsules twice daily.
- Aorta-Glycan (Enzymatic Therapy)
    One capsule twice daily.

Additional Recommendations:

- If you prefer a powdered fiber, use Fiber Plus (Yerba Prima)
    As directed.
- Hemosan (Bioforce—homeopathic)
    As directed.

Comments:

Many over-the-counter products such as suppositories, ointments, and anorectal pads used for hemorrhoids contain primarily natural ingredients, such as witch hazel, vitamin E, shark liver oil, cod liver oil, cocoa butter, Peruvian balsam, zinc oxide, live yeast cell derivative, and allantoin. However, topical therapy will only provide temporary relief in most circumstances.

HEPATITIS

Hepatitis in most instances is caused by a virus. Viral types A, B, and C are the most common. Hepatitis A occurs sporadically or in epidemics, and is transmitted primarily through fecal contamination. Hepatitis B is transmitted through infected blood or blood products. It is occasionally transmitted through saliva and sexual secretions. Hepatitis C (formerly known as hepatitis non-A, non-B) is primarily transmitted through blood transfusion. In fact, about ten percent of people receiving blood transfusions develop hepatitis C. Its incubation period is two to 20 weeks and mortality rate is unclear, but higher than for the other forms (1 to 12 percent).

Acute viral hepatitis is characterized by loss of appetite, nausea, vomiting, fatigue, and other flu-like symptoms; fever; enlarged, tender liver; jaundice (yellowing of skin due to the increased level of bilirubin in the blood); dark urine; and elevated liver enzymes in the blood. Ten percent of hepatitis B and ten to 40 percent of hepatitis C cases develop into chronic viral hepatitis forms. The symptomatology varies. The symptoms can be latent, and they can lead to chronic fatigue, serious liver damage, and even death.

Acute Hepatitis

Dietary and Lifestyle Recommendations:

• Consume vegetable broths, soups, and fresh vegetable juices.

Primary Treatment Plan:

• ThymuPlex (Enzymatic Therapy) or Thymulus (Enzymatic Therapy)
    Two tablets or two capsules twice daily.
• Super Milk Thistle (Enzymatic Therapy)
    Two capsules twice daily between meals.
• Vitamin C (any leading brand)
    500 to 1,000 mg every hour or to bowel tolerance.

Additional Recommendation:

• According to Robert Cathcart, M.D., hepatitis is "one of the easiest diseases for ascorbic acid to cure." Dr. Cathcart demonstrated that vitamin C administered intravenously at very high levels (40 g to 100 g) was able to greatly improve acute viral hepatitis in two to four days. He showed clearing of jaundice within six days. Other studies demonstrated similar benefits. For more information call or write the American College of Advancement in Medicine (ACAM), 23121 Verdugo Drive, Suite 204, Laguna Hills, CA, 92653, 1-800-532-3688 (outside California) or 1-800-435-6199 (inside California) for a referral to a physician who can prescribe weekly intravenous vitamin C therapy.

Chronic Hepatitis

Dietary and Lifestyle Recommendations:

- Consume a diet which focuses on whole, unprocessed foods (whole grains, legumes, vegetables, fruits, nuts, and seeds).
- Eliminate the intake of alcohol, caffeine, and sugar.
- Get regular exercise.
- Perform a relaxation exercise (deep breathing, meditation, prayer, visualization, etc.) for 10 to 15 minutes each day.
- Drink at least 48 ounces of water daily.

Primary Treatment Plan:

- Doctor's Choice (Male/Female) (Enzymatic Therapy)
    One tablet three times daily.
- Doctor's Choice Antioxidant Complex (Enzymatic Therapy)
    One to two tablets three times daily.
- Doctor's Choice Flax Oil Plus (Enzymatic Therapy) or Omega Twin (Barlean's)
    One tablespoon daily.
- ThymuPlex (Enzymatic Therapy) or Thymulus (Enzymatic Therapy)
    Two tablets or two capsules twice daily.
- Super Milk Thistle (Enzymatic Therapy)
    Two capsules twice daily between meals.
- Vitamin C (any leading brand)
    3,000 to 6,000 mg per day in divided dosages.

Additional Recommendations:

- Phallanthus or Eclipta Alba Herb (both by Gaia Herbs, Inc.)
    As directed.

Comments:

Thymus extracts have been shown to be effective in several double-blind studies in both acute and chronic cases. In these studies, therapeutic effect was noted by accelerated decreases of liver enzymes (transaminases), and elimination of the virus.

Country singing sensation Naomi Judd utilized natural alternatives to help her achieve remission for her hepatitis C, the most serious form of hepatitis. For more information on her story and what she did to overcome this serious illness, refer to *Health Counselor* magazine (Dec/Jan 1996).

HERPES

The Herpes simplex virus (HSV) can produce a recurrent viral infection on virtually any area of skin or mucous membranes. The most common sites are around the mouth (cold sores) and the genitals. Cold sores are usually caused by Herpes simplex virus 1 (HSV1) while genital herpes is usually caused by the type 2 virus (HSV2).

The rash in genital herpes is characterized by the appearance of single or multiple clusters of small blisters filled with a clear fluid on a reddened base. The blisters eventually burst. When they do, they leave small, painful ulcers which heal within ten to 21 days.

After the initial infection, the virus becomes dormant in the nerve root near the spine. Herpes tends to become reactivated following minor infections, trauma, and stress. The stress can be emotional, dietary, and environmental. While about 40 percent of people never have a second outbreak, others may suffer four or five attacks a year for several years or longer.

Dietary and Lifestyle Recommendations:

- Consume a diet which focuses on whole, unprocessed foods (whole grains, legumes, vegetables, and fruits).
- Avoid high arginine-containing foods (chocolate, peanuts, almonds, other nuts, and seeds).

- Eliminate the intake of alcohol, caffeine, and sugar.
- Identify and control food allergies.
- Get regular exercise.
- Perform a relaxation exercise (deep breathing, meditation, prayer, visualization, etc.) for 10 to 15 minutes each day.

Primary Treatment Plan:

- Doctor's Choice (Male/Female) (Enzymatic Therapy)
    One tablet three times daily.
- Doctor's Choice Antioxidant Complex (Enzymatic Therapy)
    One to two capsules three times daily.
- Doctor's Choice Flax Oil Plus (Enzymatic Therapy) or Omega Twin (Barlean's)
    One tablespoon daily.
- Vitamin C (any leading brand)
    3,000 mg to 8,000 mg in divided doses each day.
- ThymuPlex (Enzymatic Therapy)
    Two tablets twice daily.
- L-lysine (any leading brand)
    1,000 mg three times daily with meals.

Additional Recommendations:

- Apply Herpilyn (Enzymatic Therapy) to affected areas two to four times a day during an active recurrence. Apply it fairly thick (1 to 2 mm). Detailed toxicology studies have demonstrated that it is extremely safe and suitable for long-term use. In fact, people with recurrent cold sores should use Herpilyn on a daily basis or as soon as the first tingling sensation of a cold sore is noticed.

Comments:

Supporting and enhancing the immune system will help reduce the chance of a recurrent attack.

HIATAL HERNIA

A hiatal hernia refers to a condition in which part of the stomach extends (herniates) above the diaphragm.

Dietary and Lifestyle Recommendations:

- Do not overeat!
- Avoid chocolate and coffee.

Primary Treatment Plan:

- DGL (Enzymatic Therapy or Twin Labs)
  Two tablets twenty minutes before meals three times daily and at bedtime.
- Gastrosoothe (Enzymatic Therapy)
  Same as DGL.

Additional Recommendations:

- Elevate the head of the bed one to two inches.

Comments:

DGL will not heal the hiatal hernia, but it can greatly improve symptoms by healing the irritation of the esophagus.

HIGH BLOOD PRESSURE

A normal blood pressure reading for adults is: 120 (systolic) over 80 (diastolic). Hypertension or high blood pressure is one of the major risk factors for a heart attack or stroke. Many dietary factors have been shown to be linked with high blood pressure including:
—Obesity
—A high sodium to potassium ratio

—A diet low in fiber and high in sugar
—A diet high in saturated fats and low in essential fatty acids
—A diet low in calcium and magnesium
—A diet low in vitamin C

Dietary and Lifestyle Recommendations:

- Consume a diet which focuses on whole, unprocessed foods (whole grains, legumes, vegetables, fruits, nuts, and seeds).
- Avoid salt (sodium chloride).
- Eliminate the intake of alcohol, caffeine, and sugar.
- Get regular exercise.
- Perform a relaxation exercise (deep breathing, meditation, prayer, visualization, etc.) for 10 to 15 minutes each day.
- Drink at least 48 ounces of water daily.

Primary Treatment Plan:

- Doctor's Choice (Male/Female) (Enzymatic Therapy)
    One tablet three times daily.
- Doctor's Choice Antioxidant Complex (Enzymatic Therapy)
    One to two tablets three times daily.
- Doctor's Choice Flax Oil Plus (Enzymatic Therapy) or Omega Twin (Barlean's)
    One tablespoon daily.
- Rogenic (Enzymatic Therapy)
    Two tablets three times daily.
- Garlinase 4000 (Enzymatic Therapy)
    One tablet daily.

Additional Recommendations:

- Coenzyme Q10 (Source Naturals)
    30 to 100 mg three times daily.

Comments:

   Severe hypertension (160+ over 115+) requires immediate medical attention. A drug may be necessary to achieve initial control. Consider intravenous EDTA chelation therapy (for more information, refer to ANGINA).

HIVES

Hives or urticaria are localized swellings of the skin. Hives usually itch intensely. Hives are caused by the release of histamine within the skin. About 50 percent of patients with hives develop angioedema. This is a deeper, less-defined swelling involving tissues beneath the skin.

Hives and angioedema are relatively common conditions. It is estimated that 15 to 20 percent of the general population has had hives at some time. Although persons in any age group may experience acute or chronic hives and/or angioedema, young adults (post-adolescence through the third decade of life) are most often affected. Medications are the leading cause of hives in adults. In children, hives are usually due to foods, food additives, or infections.

Dietary and Lifestyle Recommendations:

• An elimination or low-antigenic diet is of utmost importance in the treatment of most cases of hives, particularly in children. The diet should not only eliminate suspected allergens, but also all food additives. The strictest elimination diets allow only water, lamb, rice, pears, and vegetables. Those foods most commonly associated with inducing hives (i.e. milk, eggs, chicken, fruits, nuts, and additives) should definitely be avoided.

Primary Treatment Plan:

• Doctor's Choice (Male/Female) (Enzymatic Therapy)
    One tablet three times daily.
• Doctor's Choice Antioxidant Complex (Enzymatic Therapy)
    One to two tablets three times daily.
• Doctor's Choice Flax Oil Plus (Enzymatic Therapy) or Omega Twin (Barlean's)
    One tablespoon daily.
• Quercezyme-Plus (Enzymatic Therapy)
    One to two capsules five minutes before meals. Note: Capsules can be emptied into food for infants and young children.

HOT FLASHES

(see MENOPAUSE)

HYPERACTIVITY

(see ATTENTION DEFICIT DISORDER)

HYPOGLYCEMIA

Hypoglycemia refers to a condition of low blood sugar. Because glucose is the primary fuel for the brain, when levels are too low, the brain feels the effects first. Symptoms of hypoglycemia can range from mild to severe. They include such things as: headache; depression, anxiety, irritability, and other psychological disturbances; blurred vision; excessive sweating; mental confusion; incoherent speech; bizarre behavior; and convulsions.

Conditions linked to hypoglycemia:

—Depression
—Aggressive and Criminal Behavior
—Premenstrual Syndrome
—Migraine Headaches
—Leg Cramps
—Angina

Reactive hypoglycemia is the most common type of hypoglycemia. It is characterized by the development of symptoms of hypoglycemia two to four hours after a meal.

Dietary and Lifestyle Recommendations:

- Consume a diet which focuses on whole, unprocessed foods (whole grains, legumes, vegetables, fruits, nuts, and seeds).
- Eliminate the intake of sugar, alcohol, and caffeine.
- Identify and control food allergies.
- Get regular exercise.
- Perform a relaxation exercise (deep breathing, meditation, prayer, visualization, etc.) for 10 to 15 minutes each day.
- Drink at least 48 ounces of water daily.

Primary Treatment Plan:

- Doctor's Choice (Male /Female) (Enzymatic Therapy)
    One tablet three times daily.
- Doctor's Choice Antioxidant Complex (Enzymatic Therapy)
    One to two tablets three times daily.
- Doctor's Choice Flax Oil Plus (Enzymatic Therapy) or Omega Twin (Barlean's)
    One tablespoon daily.
- Hypo-Ade (Enzymatic Therapy)
    One tablet two to three times daily with meals.

Additional Recommendations:

- Spirulina (any leading brand)
    As directed to help stabilize blood sugar levels.

HYPOTHYROIDISM

Hypothyroidism refers to a condition of an under-active thyroid gland. Common symptoms include: cold hands and feet, depression, fatigue, difficulty losing weight, poor immune function, dry skin, elevated cholesterol levels, constipation, muscle and joint stiffness, and headaches. The basal body temperature is perhaps the most sensitive functional test of thyroid function.

To determine basal body temperature:

1. Shake down the thermometer to below 95 degrees F and place it by your bed before going to sleep at night.
2. Upon waking, place the thermometer under your armpit for a full ten minutes. It is important to make as little movement as possible. Resting with your eyes closed is best. Do not get up until the ten-minute test is completed.
3. After ten minutes, read and record the temperature and date.
4. Record the temperature for at least three mornings (preferably at the same time of day) and give the information to your physician. Menstruating women must perform the test on the second, third, and fourth days of menstruation. Men and postmenopausal women can perform the test at any time.

Interpretation...

The basal body temperature should be between 97.6 and 98.2 degrees. A reading less than 97.6 degrees may indicate low thyroid.

Dietary and Lifestyle Recommendations:

- Consume a diet which focuses on whole, unprocessed foods (whole grains, legumes, vegetables, fruits, nuts, and seeds).
- Eliminate the intake of alcohol, caffeine, and sugar.
- Identify and control food allergies.
- Get regular exercise.
- Perform a relaxation exercise (deep breathing, meditation, prayer, visualization, etc.) for 10 to 15 minutes each day.
- Drink at least 48 ounces of water daily.

Primary Treatment Plan:

- Doctor's Choice (Male/Female) (Enzymatic Therapy)
    One tablet three times daily.
- Doctor's Choice Antioxidant Complex (Enzymatic Therapy)
    One to two tablets three times daily.
- Doctor's Choice Flax Oil Plus (Enzymatic Therapy) or Omega Twin (Barlean's)
    One tablespoon daily.
- Thyroid & L-Tyrosine Complex (Enzymatic Therapy)
    One or two capsules three times daily as an addition.

Additional Recommendations:

- Bladderwrack Fronds (Gaia Herbs, Inc.)
  As directed.

Comments:

Moderate to severe hypothyroidism must be treated by a prescription thyroid hormone.

IMPOTENCE

The term "impotence" has traditionally been used to signify the inability of the male to attain and maintain erection of the penis sufficient to permit satisfactory sexual intercourse. Impotence, in most circumstances, is more precisely referred to as erectile dysfunction as this term differentiates itself from loss of libido, premature ejaculation, or inability to achieve orgasm.

An estimated ten to 20 million men suffer from erectile dysfunction. This number is expected to increase dramatically as the median age of the population increases. Currently, erectile dysfunction is thought to affect over 25 percent of men over the age of 50.

Although the frequency of erectile dysfunction increases with age, it must be stressed that aging itself is not a cause of impotence. Although the amount and force of the ejaculate as well as the need to ejaculate decrease with age, the capacity for erection is retained. Men are capable of retaining their sexual virility well into their 80s.

Erectile dysfunction may be due to organic or psychogenic factors. In the overwhelming majority of cases the cause is organic, i.e., it is due to some physiological reason. In fact, in men over the age of 50, organic causes are responsible for erectile dysfunction in over 90 percent of cases. Atherosclerosis of the penile artery is the primary cause of impotence in nearly half the men over the age of 50 that have erectile dysfunction.

Dietary and Lifestyle Recommendations:

- Consume a diet which focuses on whole, unprocessed foods (whole grains, legumes, vegetables, fruits, nuts, and seeds).
- Eliminate the intake of alcohol, caffeine, and sugar.
- Identify and control food allergies.
- Get regular exercise.
- Perform a relaxation exercise (deep breathing, meditation, prayer, visualization, etc.) for 10 to 15 minutes each day.
- Drink at least 48 ounces of water daily.

Primary Treatment Plan:

- Doctor's Choice for Men (Enzymatic Therapy)
     One tablet three times daily.
- Doctor's Choice Antioxidant Complex (Enzymatic Therapy)
     One to two tablets three times daily.
- Doctor's Choice Flax Oil Plus (Enzymatic Therapy) or Omega Twin (Barlean's)
     One tablespoon daily.
- Masculex (Enzymatic Therapy)
     One or two capsules three times daily.
- Panax Ginseng Phytosome (Enzymatic Therapy)
     Two capsules in the morning.
- Ginkgo Phytosome (Enzymatic Therapy)
     One capsule three times daily before meals.

Additional Recommendations:

     If cholesterol levels are elevated, see CHOLESTEROL.
     If diabetes is a factor, see DIABETES.

Comments:

The only FDA approved medicine for impotence is yohimbine—the alkaloid isolated from the bark of the yohimbe tree (*Pausinystalia johimbe*). When used alone, yohimbine is successful in 34 to 43 percent of cases. However, side effects often make yohimbine very difficult to utilize. Yohimbine can induce anxiety, panic attacks, and hallucinations in some individuals. Other side effects include elevations in blood pressure and heart rate, dizziness, headache, and skin flushing. Yohimbine should not be used in women, individuals with kidney disease, and individuals with psychological disturbances. Because of the yohimbine content of yohimbe bark, the FDA classifies yohimbe as an unsafe herb. Because commercial sources of yohimbe bark that are available in health food stores actually state the level of yohimbine per dosage, it is difficult to determine an effective and consistent dosage.

INDIGESTION

The term "indigestion" is often used to describe a feeling of gaseousness or fullness in the abdomen. It can also be used to describe "heartburn." Indigestion can have many causes, including not only increased secretion of acid but also decreased secretion of acid and other digestive juices and enzymes.

Although most people believe that an over-acid stomach is the major cause of indigestion, a very strong case could be made for lack of gastric acid secretion being the most common reason for indigestion. Deficient production of hydrochloric acid in the stomach is known as hypochlorhydria; achlorhydria refers to a complete absence of gastric acid secretion. It is estimated that as many as 40 percent of adults may not secrete sufficient levels of hydrochloric acid, as the ability to secrete gastric acid usually decreases with age. Hypochlorhydria has been found in over half of those over age 60.

Common Symptoms, Signs, and Diseases associated with Low Hydrochloric Acid Secretion:

Symptoms
Bloating, belching, burning, and flatulence immediately after meal"
A sense of "fullness" after eating
Indigestion, diarrhea or constipation
Multiple food allergies
Nausea after taking supplements

<u>Signs</u>
Itching around the rectum
Weak, peeling and cracked fingernails
Dilated blood vessels in the cheeks and nose
Acne
Iron deficiency
Chronic intestinal parasites or abnormal flora
Undigested food in stool
Chronic candida infections
Upper digestive tract gassiness

<u>Diseases</u>
Addison's disease
Asthma
Celiac disease
Dermatitis herpetiformis
Diabetes mellitus
Eczema
Gallbladder disease
Graves' disease
Chronic auto-immune disorders
Hepatitis
Chronic hives
Lupus erythematosis
Myasthenia gravis
Osteoporosis
Pernicious anemia
Psoriasis
Rheumatoid arthritis
Rosacea
Sjogren's syndrome
Thyrotoxicosis
Hyper- and hypothyroidism
Vitiligo

Dietary and Lifestyle Recommendations:

• Chewing food thoroughly is the first step toward good digestion. Chewing signals other components of the digestive system to get ready to go to work. It also allows food to mix with saliva. Saliva contains the enzyme salivary amylase which breaks down starch molecules into smaller sugars.

Primary Treatment Plan:

• The best method of diagnosing a lack of hydrochloric acid is a special procedure known as the Heidelberg gastric analysis. This technique utilizes an electronic capsule attached to a string. The capsule is swallowed and then kept in the stomach with the aid of the string. The capsule measures the pH of the stomach and sends a radio message to a receiver which then records the pH level. The response to a bicarbonate challenge is the true test of the functional ability of the stomach to secrete acid. After the test, the capsule is pulled up from the stomach by the string attached to it. Since not everyone can have detailed gastric acid analysis to determine the need for gastric acid supplementation, a practical method of determination is often used. To determine whether you need hydrochloric acid, as well as how much your body needs for proper digestion, use the following challenge method modified from the one developed by Dr. Jonathan Wright.

1. Begin by taking one tablet of Protazyme (Enzymatic Therapy) at your next large meal. If this does not aggravate your symptoms or produce side effects like a burning sensation, pain, or gas, then at every meal after that of the same size take one more tablet. (One at the next meal, two at the meal after that, then three at the next meal.)

2. Continue to increase the dose until you reach seven tablets or when you feel a warmth in your stomach, whichever occurs first. A feeling of warmth in the stomach means that you have taken too many tablets for that meal, and you need to take one less tablet for that meal size. It is a good idea to try the larger dose again at another meal to make sure that it was the HCl that caused the warmth and not something else.

3. After you have found the largest dose that you can take at your large meals without feeling any warmth, maintain that dose at all meals of similar size. You will need to take less at smaller meals.

4. When taking a number of tablets it is best to take them throughout the meal.

5. As your stomach begins to regain the ability to produce the amount of HCl needed to properly digest your food, you will notice the warm feeling again and will have to cut down the dose level.

Additional Recommendations:

- Mega-Zyme (Enzymatic Therapy)
  Two to four tablets before meals. Pancreatic insufficiency is another common cause of indigestion.
- Digestisan (Bioforce—homeopathic)
  As directed.

Comments:

For heartburn, try GastroSoothe (Enzymatic Therapy), two to four tablets.

INFECTIONS

An infection refers to a colony of disease-causing organisms establishing a home within the body. Infections can be caused by viruses, bacteria, yeasts, and other microorganisms. The organisms actively reproduce and cause disease directly by damage to cells or indirectly by releasing toxins. It is the function of the immune system to prevent and deal with infections. Different arms of the immune system deal with different microorganisms.

Dietary and Lifestyle Recommendations:

- Rest.
- Drink plenty of liquids (focus on water, diluted vegetable juices, soups, and herb teas). Try to drink eight ounces of water every hour.
- Avoid sugar including natural sugars such as honey, orange juice, and fructose, as simple sugars depress the immune system.

Primary Treatment Plan: (Acute Viral Infections)

- ThymuPlex (Enzymatic Therapy) or Thymulus (Enzymatic Therapy)
    Two tablets or two capsules twice daily.
- EchinaFresh (Enzymatic Therapy)
    Two droppersful three times daily with glass of water.
- Vitamin C (any leading brand)
    500 to 1,000 mg every hour or to bowel tolerance.

Primary Treatment Plan: (Acute Bacterial Infections)

- Golden Spleen 500 (Enzymatic Therapy)
    Two capsules twice daily.
- Hydrastine (Enzymatic Therapy) or Golden Seal Root (Nature's Herbs)
    Two to four capsules four times daily (maximum one month at this high dosage).
- Vitamin C (any leading brand)
    500 to 1,000 mg every hour or to bowel tolerance.

INFERTILITY (Female)

Infertility in females is often a result of failure to ovulate for no apparent reason, or as a result of stress, hormonal imbalance, or a disorder of the ovary, such as a tumor or a cyst. Other, less common, causes of infertility are blocked fallopian tubes, endometriosis, or a cervical mucus which is hostile to the partner's sperm.

Dietary and Lifestyle Recommendations:

- Consume a diet which focuses on whole, unprocessed foods (whole grains, legumes, vegetables, fruits, nuts, and seeds).
- Eliminate the intake of alcohol, caffeine, and sugar.
- Identify and control food allergies.
- Get regular exercise.
- Perform a relaxation exercise (deep breathing, meditation, prayer, visualization, etc.) for 10 to 15 minutes each day.
- Drink at least 48 ounces of water daily.

Primary Treatment Plan: (for absence of ovulation)

- Doctor's Choice for Women (Enzymatic Therapy)
     One tablet three times daily.
- Doctor's Choice Antioxidant Complex (Enzymatic Therapy)
     One to two tablets three times daily.
- Doctor's Choice Flax Oil Plus (Enzymatic Therapy) or Omega Twin (Barlean's)
     One tablespoon daily.
- Chaste Berry Extract (Enzymatic Therapy)
     One or two capsules daily.
- Ovary-Uterus Complex (Enzymatic Therapy)
     One capsule three times daily.

Additional Recommendations:

- If a woman is ovulating, has no scarring and is still not conceiving, low thyroid function may be a factor. Also, the cervical mucus may be hostile. Air-Power (Enzymatic Therapy) at a dosage of two tablets three times a day may improve the fluidity of the cervical secretions.

INFERTILITY (Male)

Most causes of male infertility reflect an abnormal sperm count or quality. In about 90 percent of the cases of a low sperm count the reason is deficient sperm production. Although it only takes one sperm to fertilize an egg, in an average ejaculate a man will eject nearly 200 million sperm. However, because of the natural barriers in the female reproductive tract only about 40 or so sperm will ever reach the vicinity of an egg. There is a strong correlation between the number of sperm in an ejaculate and fertility.

Sperm formation is closely linked to nutritional and antioxidant status. Since sperm are particularly susceptible to free radical and oxidative damage, it is important that environmental sources of free radicals be avoided and the diet be rich in antioxidants.

Dietary and Lifestyle Recommendations:

- Consume a diet which focuses on whole, unprocessed foods (whole grains, legumes, vegetables, fruits, nuts, and seeds).
- Eat 1/4 cup of raw sunflower seeds or pumpkin seeds each day.
- Eliminate the intake of alcohol, caffeine, and sugar.
- Identify and control food allergies.
- Get regular exercise.
- Perform a relaxation exercise (deep breathing, meditation, prayer, visualization, etc.) for 10 to 15 minutes each day.
- Drink at least 48 ounces of water daily.

Primary Treatment Plan:

- Doctor's Choice for Men (Enzymatic Therapy)
    One tablet three times daily.
- Doctor's Choice Antioxidant Complex (Enzymatic Therapy)
    One to two capsules three times daily.
- Doctor's Choice Flax Oil Plus (Enzymatic Therapy) or Omega Twin (Barlean's)
    One tablespoon daily.
- Liquid Liver Extract with Siberian Ginseng (Enzymatic Therapy)
    One or two capsules three times daily.
- Panax Ginseng Phytosome (Enzymatic Therapy)
    Two capsules in the morning.
- Active-B12 (Enzymatic Therapy)
    One or two tablets three times daily.
- Carnitine (Enzymatic Therapy)
    300 mg three times daily.

Additional Recommendations:

The scrotal sac is supposed to keep the testes at a temperature between 94 and 96 degrees Fahrenheit. If the temperature rises above 96 degrees, sperm production is greatly inhibited or stopped completely. Typically, the mean scrotal temperature of infertile men is significantly higher than fertile men. Reducing scrotal temperature in infertile men is often enough to make them fertile. This temperature reduction is best done by not wearing tight-fitting underwear or tight jeans, avoiding hot tubs, and after exercise allowing the testicles to hang free to allow them to recover from heat buildup.

For more information, refer to Dr. Michael T. Murray's book, *Male Sexual Vitality* (part of the *Getting Well Naturally Series* from Prima Publishing, 1994) in Appendix IV of this book.

INSOMNIA

Insomnia refers to an inability to attain or maintain sleep. Over the course of a year, over one-half of the United States population will have difficulty falling asleep. About 33 percent of the population experiences insomnia on a regular basis. Foremost in the natural approach to insomnia is the elimination of those factors known to disrupt normal sleep patterns such as sources of caffeine, alcohol, and drugs.

Primary Treatment Plan: (Acute Treatment)

- Valerian Root Extract (Enzymatic Therapy)
    One or two capsules 30 to 45 minutes before retiring.
- Magnesium-Potassium Chelates (Enzymatic Therapy)
    Two tablets 30 to 45 minutes before retiring.
- Sleep Ease (Lehning Laboratories)
    20 drops in 3 ounces of water in the morning, afternoon, and just before bedtime.

Additional Recommendations:

- Melatonin (Sunsource)
  1 tablet 30 to 45 minutes before retiring is often helpful, particularly in the elderly.
- St. John's Wort Extract (Enzymatic Therapy)
  One capsule three times daily can improve sleep quality.
- KavaTone (Enzymatic Therapy)
  Three capsules 30 to 45 minutes before retiring if anxiety is contributing to insomnia.

IRRITABLE BOWEL SYNDROME

The irritable bowel syndrome (IBS) is a very common condition in which the large intestine, or colon, fails to function properly. It is also known as nervous indigestion, spastic colitis, mucous colitis, and intestinal neurosis. IBS has characteristic symptoms which can include a combination of any of the following: abdominal pain and distention, more frequent bowel movements with pain, or relief of pain with bowel movements; constipation; diarrhea; excessive production of mucus in the colon; symptoms of indigestion such as flatulence, nausea, or anorexia; and varying degrees of anxiety or depression. IBS is an extremely common condition. Estimates suggest that approximately 15 percent of the population have suffered from IBS.

Dietary and Lifestyle Recommendations:

- Consume a diet which focuses on whole, unprocessed foods (whole grains, legumes, vegetables, fruits, nuts, and seeds).
- Eliminate the intake of alcohol, caffeine, and sugar.
- Identify and control food allergies.
- Get regular exercise.
- Perform a relaxation exercise (deep breathing, meditation, prayer, visualization, etc.) for 10 to 15 minutes each day.
- Drink at least 48 ounces of water daily.

Primary Treatment Plan:

- Doctor's Choice (Male/Female) (Enzymatic Therapy)
  One tablet three times daily.
- Doctor's Choice Antioxidant Complex (Enzymatic Therapy)
  One to two capsules three times daily.
- Doctor's Choice Flax Oil Plus (Enzymatic Therapy) or Omega Twin (Barlean's)
  One to two tablespoons daily.
- Peppermint Plus (Enzymatic Therapy)
  One or two capsules twice daily between meals.
- Enzydophilus (Enzymatic Therapy)
  One capsule three times daily with meals for the first week.
  Thereafter, one capsule daily with a meal.
- Dietary Fiber (Enzymatic Therapy)
  Two to four capsules at night before going to bed.

Additional Recommendations:

- Candida Formula (Enzymatic Therapy)
  One or two capsules twice daily between meals.

Comments:

Avoiding white sugar, consuming a diet rich in complex carbohydrates and dietary fiber, and eliminating food allergies is effective in most cases.

KIDNEY STONES

In the United States, most kidney stones are calcium-containing stones composed of calcium oxalate, calcium oxalate mixed with calcium phosphate, or, very rarely, calcium phosphate alone. The high rate of calcium-containing stones in affluent societies is directly associated with the following dietary patterns: low fiber, highly refined carbohydrates, high alcohol consumption, large amounts of animal protein, high fat, high calcium-containing food, high salt, and high vitamin D enriched food.

Dietary and Lifestyle Recommendations:

- Consume a diet which focuses on whole, unprocessed foods (whole grains, legumes, vegetables, fruits, nuts, and seeds).
- Eliminate the intake of antacids, alcohol, caffeine, and sugar.
- Drink at least 48 ounces of water daily.

Primary Treatment Plan:

- Doctor's Choice (Male/Female) (Enzymatic Therapy)
    One tablet three times daily.
- Doctor's Choice Antioxidant Complex (Enzymatic Therapy)
    One to two capsules three times daily.
- Doctor's Choice Flax Oil Plus (Enzymatic Therapy) or Omega Twin (Barlean's)
    One to two tablespoons daily.
- CranExtra (Enzymatic Therapy) or Aqua-Flow (Enzymatic Therapy)
    One to two capsules three times daily with a glass of water.
- Magnesium-Potassium Chelate (Enzymatic Therapy)
    One tablet three times daily.

Additional Recommendations:

- Acid-A-Cal (Enzymatic Therapy)
    As directed.
- Fresh Gravel Root (Gaia Herbs, Inc.)
    As directed.

LUPUS

Lupus most often refers to Systemic Lupus Erythematosus, a condition which affects many systems of the body, including the skin, joints and kidneys. Lupus is a classic example of an autoimmune type disease in which the body's immune system attacks connective tissue. Lupus affects women nine times more often than men. Lupus is life-threatening when the kidneys become involved.

Dietary and Lifestyle Recommendations:

- Consume a diet which focuses on whole, unprocessed foods (whole grains, legumes, vegetables, fruits, nuts, and seeds).
- Avoid animal products with the exception of cold water fish (salmon, mackerel, herring, halibut, etc.).
- Identify and control food allergies.
- Eliminate the intake of alcohol, caffeine, and sugar.
- Get regular exercise.
- Perform a relaxation exercise (deep breathing, meditation, prayer, visualization, etc.) for 10 to 15 minutes each day.
- Drink at least 48 ounces of water daily.

Primary Treatment Plan:

- Doctor's Choice (Male/Female) (Enzymatic Therapy)
      One tablet three times daily.
- Doctor's Choice Antioxidant Complex (Enzymatic Therapy)
      One to two capsules three times daily.
- Doctor's Choice Flax Oil Plus (Enzymatic Therapy) or Omega Twin (Barlean's)
      One to two tablespoons daily.
- Mega-Zyme (Enzymatic Therapy)
      Two to four tablets twice daily between meals.
- Adrenal-Cortex Complex (Enzymatic Therapy)
      One to three capsules daily.
- Curazyme (Enzymatic Therapy)
      Two to four tablets twice daily between meals.

Additional Recommendations:

- If corticosteroids have been used at either high dosages or long-term, recommend Raw Adrenal (Enzymatic Therapy) and/or Adren-Comp (Enzymatic Therapy).

LYME DISEASE

Lyme disease is characterized by skin changes, flu-like symptoms, and joint inflammation. It was first described in the community of Old Lyme, CT, in 1975. Lyme disease is caused by a bacterium (*Borrelia burgdorferi*) that is transmitted by the bite of a tick that usually lives on deer but can infest dogs. In the acute stage, Lyme disease is best treated with antibiotics to prevent the development of the chronic inflammatory condition. The following dosages are for the chronic form.

Dietary and Lifestyle Recommendations:

- Consume a diet which focuses on whole, unprocessed foods (whole grains, legumes, vegetables, fruits, nuts, and seeds).
- Avoid animal products with the exception of cold water fish (salmon, mackerel, herring, halibut, etc.).
- Identify and control food allergies.
- Eliminate the intake of alcohol, caffeine, and sugar.
- Get regular exercise.
- Perform a relaxation exercise (deep breathing, meditation, prayer, visualization, etc.) for 10 to 15 minutes each day.
- Drink at least 48 ounces of water daily.

Primary Treatment Plan:

- Doctor's Choice (Male/Female) (Enzymatic Therapy)
    One tablet three times daily.
- Doctor's Choice Antioxidant Complex (Enzymatic Therapy)
    One to two capsules three times daily.
- Doctor's Choice Flax Oil Plus (Enzymatic Therapy) or Omega Twin (Barlean's)
    One to two tablespoons daily.
- Mega-Zyme (Enzymatic Therapy)
    Two to four tablets twice daily between meals.
- Adrenal-Cortex Complex (Enzymatic Therapy)
    One to three capsules daily.
- Curazyme (Enzymatic Therapy)
    Two to four tablets twice daily between meals.

Additional Recommendations:

If corticosteroids have been used at either high dosages or long-term, try Raw Adrenal (Enzymatic Therapy) and/or Adren-Comp (Enzymatic Therapy).

MACULAR DEGENERATION

The macula is the portion of the eye responsible for fine vision. Degeneration of the macula is the leading cause of severe vision loss in the United States and Europe in persons aged 55 years or older. The risk factors for macular degeneration include aging, atherosclerosis, and high blood pressure. There is no current medical treatment for the most common form of macular degeneration. Laser surgery is used for those individuals who develop a less common type of macular degeneration (exudative macular degeneration).

The origin of macular degeneration is ultimately related to damage caused by free radicals. As with most diseases related to free radical damage, prevention or treatment at an early stage is more effective than trying to reverse the disease process.

Dietary and Lifestyle Recommendations:

- Consume a diet which focuses on whole, unprocessed foods (whole grains, legumes, vegetables, fruits, nuts, and seeds).
- Eliminate the intake of alcohol, caffeine, and sugar.
- Get regular exercise.
- Perform a relaxation exercise (deep breathing, meditation, prayer, visualization, etc.) for 10 to 15 minutes each day.
- Drink at least 48 ounces of water daily.

Primary Treatment Plan:

- Doctor's Choice (Male/Female) (Enzymatic Therapy)
    One tablet three times daily.

- Doctor's Choice Antioxidant Complex (Enzymatic Therapy)
  One to two capsules three times daily.
- Doctor's Choice Flax Oil Plus (Enzymatic Therapy) or Omega Twin (Barlean's)
  One to two tablespoons daily.
- Ginkgo Phytosome (Enzymatic Therapy) and/or Bilberry Extract
  (Enzymatic Therapy)
  One capsule three times daily.
- Cata-Comp (Enzymatic Therapy)
  One or two capsules three times daily.

Additional Recommendations:

- Eyebright Combination (BioForce)
  Two drops in each eye per night, do not open eye for 1/2 hour.

Comments:

Numerous studies have shown that individuals consuming more fruits and vegetables are less likely to develop cataracts or macular degeneration compared to individuals who do not regularly consume fruits and vegetables. Fresh fruits and vegetables are rich in a broad range of antioxidant compounds including vitamin C, carotenes, flavonoids, and glutathione. All of these antioxidants are critically involved in important mechanisms which prevent the development of macular degeneration.

MENOPAUSE

Menopause denotes the cessation of menstruation in women. It usually occurs when a woman reaches the age of fifty. Six to twelve months without a period is the commonly accepted rule for diagnosing menopause. The time period prior to the official designation of menopause is often referred to as "perimenopausal" while the time period after menopause is officially diagnosed is referred to as post-menopausal.

Menopause is currently viewed more as a disease rather than a normal physiological process. Current medical treatment of menopause primarily involves the use of hormone replacement therapy featuring the combination of estrogen and progesterone. However, this treatment carries with it significant risk and side effects, such as headache, fatigue, depression, vaginal candidiasis, breast tenderness, or skin problems. In addition, according to the *Physician's Desk Reference*, studies have linked long-term usage of estrogen with an increased risk of breast cancer. Estrogens have also been reported to increase the risk of endometrial cancer in postmenopausal women.

Dietary and Lifestyle Recommendations:

- Consume a diet which focuses on whole, unprocessed foods (whole grains, legumes, vegetables, fruits, nuts, and seeds).
- Increase consumption of soy foods.
- Eliminate the intake of alcohol, caffeine, and sugar.
- Get regular exercise.
- Perform a relaxation exercise (deep breathing, meditation, prayer, visualization, etc.) for 10 to 15 minutes each day.
- Drink at least 48 ounces of water daily.

Primary Treatment Plan:

- Doctor's Choice for Women—Senior Formula (Enzymatic Therapy)
    One tablet three times daily.
- Doctor's Choice Antioxidant Complex (Enzymatic Therapy)
    One to two capsules three times daily.
- OsteoPrime (Enzymatic Therapy)
    Two capsules.
- Doctor's Choice Flax Oil Plus (Enzymatic Therapy) or Omega Twin (Barlean's)
    One to two tablespoons daily.
- Remifemin (Enzymatic Therapy)
    Two tablets twice daily.

Additional Recommendations:

- Femtrol (Enzymatic Therapy) can also be used to reduce symptoms of hot flashes and vaginal atrophy. If there is anxiety as a menopausal symptom, add Kava-Tone (Enzymatic Therapy) to the supplement protocol.
- Menosan (Bioforce—homeopathic)
    As directed.

Comments:

For more information refer to Dr. Michael T. Murray's book, *Menopause* (part of the *Getting Well Naturally Series* from Prima Publishing, 1994) listed in Appendix IV of this book.

MENSTRUAL DISORDERS

(see appropriate topic, e.g., INFERTILITY, FIBROCYSTIC BREAST DISEASE, or PREMENSTRUAL SYNDROME)

MIGRAINE HEADACHE

Migraine headaches are vascular headaches characterized by throbbing pain, which pounds sharply in the head of the sufferer. In contrast, a tension headache is associated with a steady, constant pain that starts at the forehead or back of head and can spread pain over the entire head. Sometimes migraines hit without warning. Many who suffer migraines get unusual symptoms called "auras" before the pain hits. The aura may be a tingling or numbness in the body. Alternatively, the individual's vision may become blurred or show bright spots. Thinking may become disturbed. Anxiety or fatigue may suddenly occur. A surprisingly high percentage of Americans suffer from migraines. The percentage is higher for women (25 percent to 30 percent) than for men (14 percent to 20 percent). A family history of the illness is discovered with more than half of the sufferers.

Dietary and Lifestyle Recommendations:

- Consume a diet which focuses on whole, unprocessed foods (whole grains, legumes, vegetables, fruits, nuts, and seeds).
- Avoid animal products with the exception of cold water fish (salmon, mackerel, herring, halibut, etc.).
- Identify and control food allergies.

- Eliminate the intake of alcohol, caffeine, and sugar.
- Get regular exercise.
- Perform a relaxation exercise (deep breathing, meditation, prayer, visualization, etc.) for 10 to 15 minutes each day.
- Drink at least 48 ounces of water daily.

Primary Treatment Plan:

- Doctor's Choice (Male/Female) (Enzymatic Therapy)
    One tablet three times daily.
- Doctor's Choice Antioxidant Complex (Enzymatic Therapy)
    One to two capsules three times daily.
- Doctor's Choice Flax Oil Plus (Enzymatic Therapy) or Omega Twin (Barlean's)
    One tablespoon daily.
- Mygracare (Enzymatic Therapy)
    One capsule daily.
- Gingerall (Enzymatic Therapy)
    One to three capsules daily.
- Magnesium-Potassium Chelate (Enzymatic Therapy)
    One tablet three times daily.

Additional Recommendations:

- Rule out hypothyroidism, as hypothyroidism can be associated with a tendency toward migraine headaches.
- Migrainosan (Bioforce—homeopathic)
    As directed.

Comments:

A recent analysis of the parthenolide content of over 35 different commercial preparations indicate a wide variation in the amount of parthenolide. Mygracare (Enzymatic Therapy) is standardized to contain 600 mcg of parthenolide per capsule.

MONONUCLEOSIS

(see INFECTIONS)

MULTIPLE SCLEROSIS

Multiple sclerosis (MS) is a syndrome of progressive nervous system disturbances occurring early in life. The early symptoms of multiple sclerosis may include:

Muscular symptoms—Feeling of heaviness, weakness, leg dragging, stiffness, tendency to drop things, clumsiness

Sensory symptoms—Tingling, "pins and needles" sensation, numbness, dead feeling, band-like tightness, electrical sensations

Visual symptoms—Blurring, fogginess, haziness, eyeball pain, blindness, double vision

Vestibular symptoms—Light-headedness, feeling of spinning, sensation of drunkenness, nausea, vomiting

Genitourinary symptoms—Incontinence, loss of bladder sensation, loss of sexual function

Despite considerable research, there are still many questions about MS. Mainstream medicine has become almost obsessed with finding a viral cause for this disease, although most current work suggests immune disturbances. In MS, the myelin sheath that surrounds nerves is destroyed. For this reason MS is classified as a "demyelinating" disease. Zones of demyelination (plaques) vary in size and location within the spinal cord. Symptoms correspond in a general way to the distribution of the plaques.

In about two-thirds of the cases, onset is between ages 20 and 40 (rarely is the onset after 50) and females are affected slightly more often than males (60 percent female:40 percent male). The cause of MS remains to be definitively determined. Many causative factors have been proposed including viruses, autoimmune factors, and diet.

Dietary and Lifestyle Recommendations:

- Consume a diet which focuses on whole, unprocessed foods (whole grains, legumes, vegetables, fruits, nuts, and seeds).
- Avoid animal products with the exception of cold water fish (salmon, mackerel, herring, halibut, etc.).
- Identify and control food allergies.
- Eliminate the intake of alcohol, caffeine, and sugar.
- Get regular exercise.
- Perform a relaxation exercise (deep breathing, meditation, prayer, visualization, etc.) for 10 to 15 minutes each day.
- Drink at least 48 ounces of water daily.

Primary Treatment Plan:

- Doctor's Choice (Male/Female) (Enzymatic Therapy)
    One tablet three times daily.
- Doctor's Choice Antioxidant Complex (Enzymatic Therapy)
    Two capsules three times daily.
- Doctor's Choice Flax Oil Plus (Enzymatic Therapy) or Omega Twin (Barlean's)
    One or two tablespoons daily.
- Ginkgo Phytosome (Enzymatic Therapy)
    One capsule three times daily.
- Mega-Zyme (Enzymatic Therapy)
    Two to four tablets twice daily between meals.

Additional Recommendations:

- Grape Seed (PCO) Phytosome (Enzymatic Therapy)
    One capsule three times daily.

Comments:

Dr. Roy Swank, Professor of Neurology, University of Oregon Medical School, has provided convincing evidence that a diet low in saturated fats, maintained over a long period of time (one study lasted over 34 years), tends to halt the disease process. Swank began successfully treating patients with his low-fat diet in 1948. Swank's diet recommends: (1) a saturated fat intake of no more than 10 grams per day; (2) a daily intake of 40 to 50 grams of polyunsaturated oils (margarine, shortening, and hydrogenated oils are not allowed); (3) at least 1 tsp. of cod liver oil daily; (4) a normal allowance of protein; and (5) the consumption of fish three or more times a week.

OSTEOARTHRITIS

Osteoarthritis or degenerative joint disease is the most common form of arthritis. It is seen primarily, but not exclusively, in the elderly. Surveys have indicated that over 40 million Americans have osteoarthritis, including 80 percent of persons over the age of 50. Under the age of 45, osteoarthritis is much more common in men; after age 45 it is ten times more common in women than men.

The weight-bearing joints and joints of the hands are the joints most often affected by the degenerative changes associated with osteoarthritis. Specifically, there is much cartilage destruction followed by hardening and the formation of large bone spurs in the joint margins. Pain, deformity, and limitation of motion in the joint results. Inflammation is usually minimal.

The onset of osteoarthritis can be very subtle; morning joint stiffness is often the first symptom. As the disease progresses, there is pain on motion of the involved joint that is made worse by prolonged activity and relieved by rest. There is usually no sign of inflammation.

Dietary and Lifestyle Recommendations:

- Consume a diet which focuses on whole, unprocessed foods (whole grains, legumes, vegetables, fruits, nuts, and seeds).
- Avoid animal products with the exception of cold water fish (salmon, mackerel, herring, halibut, etc.).
- Identify and control food allergies.
- Eliminate the intake of alcohol, caffeine, and sugar.
- Get regular exercise. If weight-bearing joints are severely affected activities such as swimming, water aerobics, and bike riding should be encouraged.
- Perform a relaxation exercise (deep breathing, meditation, prayer, visualization, etc.) for 10 to 15 minutes each day.
- Drink at least 48 ounces of water daily.

(continued on page 120)

Osteoarthritis:
Glucosamine sulfate vs. NAG

To clarify the difference between glucosamine sulfate and other forms of glucosamine, we decided to ask leading natural medicine researcher, Dr. Michael Murray, several questions.

Q. Dr. Murray, companies selling N-acetyl-glucosamine, commonly referred to as "NAG," have stated in product literature that NAG is better absorbed, more stable, and is better utilized than glucosamine sulfate. What are your feelings regarding these claims?

Dr. Murray: These contentions are without support in the scientific literature. Glucosamine sulfate is clearly the preferred form. Detailed human studies on the absorption, distribution, and elimination of orally administered glucosamine sulfate have shown an absorption rate of as high as 98 percent and that once absorbed it is then distributed primarily to joint tissues where it is incorporated into the connective tissue matrix of cartilage, ligaments, and tendons (Setnikar I, et al. Arzneim Forsch 36:729, 1986; Setnikar I, et al. Arzneim Forsch 43:1109, 1993). In addition, there have been over 20 double-blind placebo-controlled studies on glucosamine sulfate as a nutritional aid to humans. In contrast, to my knowledge, there has never been a double-blind study using NAG for any application. Nor have there ever been any detailed absorption studies on NAG in humans.

Further evidence of the superiority of glucosamine sulfate to NAG is offered by studies in laboratory animals. Over the years, numerous researchers (e.g., Capps JC, et al. Biochim Biophys Acta 127:194, 1966; Kohn P, et al. J Biol Chem 237:304, 1962; Richmond JE. Biochemistry 2:676, 1963; McGarrahan JF, et al. J Biol Chem 224:649, 1957; and Lefevre J, Gen Physiol 31:505, 1948) have demonstrated that glucosamine is superior to NAG in terms of absorption and utilization by at least a factor of 2:1. These researchers have concluded that glucosamine is a more efficient precursor of macromolecular hexosamine [glycosaminoglycans] than N-acetylglucosamine. It is possible that N-acetylglucosamine does not penetrate the cell membranes and, as a result, is not available for incorporation into glycoproteins and mucopolysaccharides. (Note see: Capps JC, et al. Biochim Biophys Acta 127:205, 1966).

Q. Are you saying that the body may not absorb NAG?

Dr. Murray: The absorption of NAG is questionable in humans for several reasons: (1) NAG is quickly digested by intestinal bacteria; (2) NAG is a known binder of dietary lectins in the gut with the resultant lectin-NAG complex being excreted in the feces; and (3) a large percentage of NAG is broken down by intestinal cells (Capps JC, et al. Biochim Biophys Acta 127:194, 1966).

Q. How is NAG different from glucosamine sulfate?

Dr. Murray: NAG differs from glucosamine sulfate in that instead of a sulfur molecule, NAG has a portion of an acetic acid molecule attached to it. Glucosamine sulfate and NAG are entirely different molecules and appear to be handled by the body differently. The body preferentially utilizes glucosamine sulfate compared to NAG. This preference is exhibited by the fact that the absorption of glucosamine sulfate is an active process. In other words, there are mechanisms in the body which are designed specifically for the absorption and utilization of glucosamine sulfate. No such mechanisms exist for NAG (Tesoriere G, et al. Experentia 28:770, 1972).

Q. Another form of glucosamine that is now being marketed is glucosamine hydrochloride. What are your opinions on this form?

Dr. Murray: As with NAG, the research simply does not support the use of glucosamine hydrochloride. It appears that the sulfur component of glucosamine sulfate may be critical to the beneficial effects noted. Sulfur is an essential nutrient for joint tissue where it functions in the stabilization of the connective tissue matrix of cartilage, tendons, and ligaments. As far back as the 1930s and 1940s, researchers demonstrated that individuals with arthritis are commonly deficient in this essential nutrient. Restoring sulfur levels brought about significant benefit to these patients. Therefore, it appears the sulfur portion of glucosamine sulfate is extremely important and is another reason why glucosamine sulfate is the preferred form of glucosamine.

Q. How important is it that people with osteoarthritis use the proper form of glucosamine?

Dr. Murray: In order for people to gain the benefit from many natural products, they must use the right form. If people with osteoarthritis want to gain the benefits of glucosamine noted in the scientific studies, they had better make sure they are taking 500 mg of glucosamine sulfate three times daily.

Primary Treatment Plan:

- Doctor's Choice (Male/Female) (Enzymatic Therapy)
    One tablet three times daily.
- Doctor's Choice Antioxidant Complex (Enzymatic Therapy)
    Two capsules three times daily.
- Doctor's Choice Flax Oil Plus (Enzymatic Therapy) or Omega Twin (Barlean's)
    One or two tablespoons daily.
- Armax (Enzymatic Therapy)
    Two tablets three times daily with meals.
- Arthritis Formula (Lehning Laboratories)
    One tablespoon in morning and at bedtime.
- Artho-Soothe (Enzymatic Therapy)
    Apply to affected areas twice daily.

Additional Recommendations:

- If there is inflammation, take Gingerall (Enzymatic Therapy) at a dosage of one capsule three times daily or Curazyme (Enzymatic Therapy) two to four capsules twice daily between meals. If there are calcium deposits (especially in the spine), take Acid-A-Cal (Enzymatic Therapy) at a dosage of two capsules with meals and at bedtime (four times daily).
- Arthritisan (Bioforce—homeopathic)
    As directed.

Comments:

Armax provides not only glucosamine sulfate, but other nutrients critical to healthy joint function.

OSTEOPOROSIS

Osteoporosis literally means porous bone. Osteoporosis affects more than 20 million people in the United States. Normally there is a decline in bone mass after the age of 40 in both sexes. This bone loss is accelerated in patients with osteoporosis. Many factors can result in excessive bone loss and different variants of osteoporosis exist. Postmenopausal osteoporosis in women is the most common form of osteoporosis.

Major Risk Factors for Osteoporosis in Women:

Postmenopausal
White or Asian
Premature menopause
Positive family history
Short stature and small bones
Leanness
Low calcium intake
Inactivity
Nulliparity (never pregnant)
Gastric or small-bowel resection
Long-term glucocorticosteroid therapy
Long-term use of anticonvulsants
Hyperparathyroidism
Hyperthyroidism
Smoking
Heavy alcohol use

To determine if you are at risk for osteoporosis, complete the questionnaire on pages 122 and 123.

Dietary and Lifestyle Recommendations:

• Consume a diet which focuses on whole, unprocessed foods (whole grains, legumes, vegetables, fruits, nuts, and seeds).
• Eliminate the intake of alcohol, caffeine, and sugar.
• Do not drink soft drinks.
• Get regular exercise.
• Walk!
• Perform a relaxation exercise (deep breathing, meditation, prayer, visualization, etc.) for 10 to 15 minutes each day.
• Drink at least 48 ounces of water daily.

(continued on page 124)

Osteoporosis:
Are you at risk?

Choose the item in each category that best describes you, and fill in the point value for that item in the space at the right. You may choose more than one item in categories marked with an asterisk.

	Points	Score
Frame size		
Small-boned or petite	10	
Medium frame, very lean	5	
Medium frame, average or heavy build	0	
Large frame, very lean	5	
Ethnic Background		
Caucasian	10	
Asian	10	
Other	0	
Activity Level		
How often do you walk briskly, jog, engage in aerobics, or perform hard physical labor, of a duration of at least 30 minutes?		
Seldom	30	
1-2 times per week	20	
3-4 times per week	5	
5 or more times per week	0	
Smoking		
Smoke 10 or more cigarettes a day	20	
Smoke fewer than 10 cigarettes a day	10	
Quit smoking	5	
Never smoked	0	
Personal Health Factors*		
Family history of osteoporosis	20	
Long-term corticosteroid use	20	
Long-term anticonvulsant use	20	

Drink more than 3 glasses of alcohol per week	20
Drink more than one cup of coffee per day	10
Seldom get outside in the sun	10
Had ovaries removed	10
Premature menopause	10
Had no children	10

Dietary Factors*

Consume more than 4 ounces of meat on a daily basis	20
Drink soft drinks regularly	20
Consume 3-5 servings of vegetables per day	-10
Consume at least one cup of green leafy vegetables each day	-10
Take a calcium supplement	-10
Consume a vegetarian diet	-10

Total Score

Interpretation

If the score is higher than 50, the patient is at significant risk for osteoporosis. Hormonal replacement may be suitable for these patients, especially if they experienced an early menopause, had their ovaries surgically removed, or never had children.

Before initiating hormone replacement therapy, it is important to reduce the risk factors that a patient can control such as starting an exercise program; quitting smoking; not drinking alcohol, coffee, or soft drinks; taking a good calcium supplement; and consuming a diet low in protein and high in vegetables. These changes could take as many as 150 points off the patient's score, possibly eliminating the risk for osteoporosis.

Since both estrogen and progesterone have been shown to exert beneficial effects against bone loss and actually increase bone mass, estrogen-progesterone combinations are preferred to estrogen alone. The exception is in women at high risk for breast cancer or women with a disease aggravated by estrogen including breast cancer, active liver diseases, and certain cardiovascular diseases, in which case progesterone alone should be used.

Primary Treatment Plan:

- Doctor's Choice for Women (Enzymatic Therapy)
  One tablet three times daily.
- Doctor's Choice Antioxidant Complex (Enzymatic Therapy)
  Two capsules three times daily.
- Doctor's Choice Flax Oil Plus (Enzymatic Therapy) or Omega Twin (Barlean's)
  One or two tablespoons daily.
- OsteoPrime (Enzymatic Therapy)
  Two tablets twice daily.
- Remifemin (Enzymatic Therapy)
  Two tablets twice daily (if postmenopausal).

Additional Recommendations:

- Ionized Calcium with Magnesium (Enzymatic Therapy) or Calcium-Magnesium Chelate (Enzymatic Therapy)
  One tablet or capsule three times daily.

Comments:

For more information on osteoporosis refer to *Preventing and Reversing Osteoporosis* by Alan R. Gaby, M.D., listed in Appendix IV of this book.

PARASITES (INTESTINAL)

A parasite is any organism living in or on any other living creature. When people refer to "intestinal parasites," most often they are loosely referring to single-celled organisms known as protozoa (such as giardia and amoeba). However, strictly speaking, all organisms in the intestinal tract are parasites, even the health promoting bacteria like L. acidophilus. Because of the seriousness of some untreated protozoal infection, customers should be directed to a physician if they are experiencing symptoms of violent attacks of diarrhea, severe abdominal discomfort, and fever.

Primary Treatment Plan:

- Parazyme (Enzymatic Therapy)
  Two capsules three times daily with meals.
- Mega-Zyme (Enzymatic Therapy)
  Four tablets three times daily between meals.
- Hydrastine (Enzymatic Therapy)
  Four capsules three times daily between meals.
- Enzydophilus (Enzymatic Therapy)
  One capsule three times daily with meals for the first week.
  Thereafter, one capsule daily with a meal.

Additional Recommendations:

- Grapefruit Seed Extract (Nutribiotics)
  As directed.

Comments:

For more information on parasites, refer to Ann Louise Gittleman's book, *Guess What Came to Dinner*, listed in Appendix IV of this book.

PARKINSON'S DISEASE

Parkinson's disease is a disorder in the brain that causes muscle tremor, weakness, and stiffness. The characteristic signs are trembling, a rigid posture, slow movements, and a shuffling, unbalanced walk. Parkinson's disease is caused by degeneration of nerve cells due largely to free radical damage. In all but the initial phase of the disease, drug therapy is necessary.

Dietary and Lifestyle Recommendations:

- Consume a diet which focuses on whole, unprocessed foods (whole grains, legumes, vegetables, fruits, nuts, and seeds).
- Eliminate the intake of alcohol, caffeine, and sugar.
- Get regular exercise.

- Perform a relaxation exercise (deep breathing, meditation, prayer, visualization, etc.) for 10 to 15 minutes each day.
- Drink at least 48 ounces of water daily.

Primary Treatment Plan:

- Doctor's Choice (Male/Female) (Enzymatic Therapy)
      One tablet three times daily.
- Doctor's Choice Antioxidant Complex (Enzymatic Therapy)
      Two capsules three times daily.
- Doctor's Choice Flax Oil Plus (Enzymatic Therapy) or Omega Twin (Barlean's)
      One or two tablespoons daily.
- Carotene Complex (Enzymatic Therapy)
      One or two capsules daily.

Parkinson's Disease:
Nutrient treatment results quite promising.

Clinical studies regarding the treatment of Parkinson's disease with vitamins C and E provide new hope for slowing down the progression of this disease.

According to the *Vital Communications Natural Medicine Update* by Dr. Michael T. Murray, pilot studies beginning in 1979 evaluated 21 patients with Parkinson's disease. For a period of seven years the patients were given 3,000 mg of vitamin C and 3,200 IU of vitamin E daily.

Although all of the patients required drug therapy, the progression of the disease as determined by the need for medication was considerably delayed in those receiving the vitamins.

Dr. Murray concluded, "These results are quite promising... Perhaps more effective antioxidant combinations will provide even greater benefit."

Parkinson's disease is a brain disorder which causes muscle tremors, stiffness, and weakness. It is characterized by trembling, a rigid posture, slow movements, and a shuffling, unbalanced walk. The cause of Parkinson's disease is presently unknown.

—*Vital Communications Natural Medicine Update* by Michael T. Murray, N.D., Vol. 1, No. 5.

- Ginkgo Phytosome (Enzymatic Therapy)
    One capsule three times daily.
- Grape Seed (PCO) Phytosome (Enzymatic Therapy)
    One capsule two to three times daily.

Additional Recommendations:

- Phosphatidylserine (Enzymatic Therapy)
    100 mg three times daily.
- Rule out heavy metal toxicity by performing a hair mineral analysis.

Comments:

About one-third of individuals with Parkinson's disease go on to develop dementia. Ginkgo biloba extract has been shown to be effective in halting this progression.

PERIODONTAL DISEASE AND GINGIVITIS

Periodontal disease is characterized by localized pain of the gum tissue, loose teeth, dental pockets, redness, swelling and/or pus, or jaw bone destruction. Periodontal disease usually begins as gingivitis, which is inflammation, redness, and/or bleeding of the gums. There are a variety of things that can cause periodontal disease including, but not limited to:
- bacterial plaque
- a weak immune system
- faulty dental fillings
- tobacco smoking
- connective tissue and collagen weakness

It is estimated that 80 percent to 90 percent of the American population has some degree of periodontal disease. Contrary to popular belief or reality, your teeth should last a lifetime. Yet a large percentage of Americans are wearing dentures by the time they are 45 years old.

Lifestyle and Dietary Recommendations:

- Proper oral hygiene is a must if you wish to prevent periodontal disease. Regular brushing, flossing and dental check-ups and cleanings should be a part of your oral hygiene program.
- Avoid eating sugary foods. A natural diet featuring as few unprocessed foods as possible is the best.

Primary Treatment Plan:

- Doctor's Choice (Male/Female) (Enzymatic Therapy)
    One tablet three times daily.
- Doctor's Choice Antioxidant Formula (Enzymatic Therapy)
    Two capsules times daily
- Ultra Co-Q10 (Twin Labs)
    100 mg capsules
- Oral Basics (Enzymatic Therapy)
    Provides specific vitamins and minerals essential for healthy gums.

Additional Recommendations: (Acute Phase)

- Zinc (any leading brand)
    Extra zinc in the diet will fight free radicals, stabilize membranes, synthesize collagen, inhibit plaque growth, and stimulate immune function.
- Vira-Plex (Enzymatic Therapy)
    Contains extra nutrients, including vitamin A, that will help alleviate infection in the gums.
- Vitamin C (any leading brand)
    Additional vitamin C will help reduce inflammation, stimulate the immune system, and heal gum tissue. Take until bowel tolerance. Keep in mind that very high doses of vitamin C can cause loose bowels and cramping.

PLEURISY

(see BRONCHITIS and PNEUMONIA)

PREMENSTRUAL SYNDROME

Premenstrual syndrome (PMS), also called premenstrual tension, is a recurrent condition of women characterized by troublesome, yet often ill-defined, symptoms seven to 14 days before menstruation. Typical symptoms include: decreased energy, tension, irritability, depression, headache, altered sex drive, breast pain, backache, abdominal bloating, and swelling of the fingers and ankles. The syndrome affects about one-third of women between 30 and 40 years of age, about ten percent of whom may have a significantly debilitating form.

Although there is a wide spectrum of symptoms, there are common hormonal patterns in PMS patients when compared to symptom free control groups. Perhaps the most common pattern is an elevation of plasma estrogen and a decrease in plasma progesterone levels five to ten days before the menses.

Dietary and Lifestyle Recommendations:

Diet appears to play a major role in the development of PMS. Compared to symptom-free women, PMS patients consume: 62 percent more refined carbohydrates, 275 percent more refined sugar, 79 percent more dairy products, 78 percent more sodium, 53 percent less iron, 77 percent less manganese and 52 percent less zinc. The first step in addressing PMS is to limit the consumption of refined sugar and decrease or eliminate milk and dairy products.

Additional key dietary recommendations for the PMS sufferer include decreasing salt intake, alcohol and tobacco use, and the intake of caffeine-containing foods and beverages such as coffee, tea, and chocolate. Caffeine intake has been shown to produce a dose-dependent effect on the severity of symptoms, i.e., the more caffeine consumed, the greater the severity of the symptoms.

Primary Treatment Plan:

- Doctor's Choice for Women (Enzymatic Therapy)
  One tablet three times daily.
- Doctor's Choice Antioxidant Complex (Enzymatic Therapy)
  One to two capsules three times daily.
- Doctor's Choice Flax Oil Plus (Enzymatic Therapy) or Omega Twin (Barlean's)
  One to two tablespoons daily.
- Female Balance (Enzymatic Therapy)
  Three to six capsules daily during periods of PMS.
- Female Relief (Lehning Laboratories)
  20 drops in 3 ounces of water every four hours, three times a day.

Additional Recommendations:

- For general hormonal support, try one of the following: Remifemin (Enzymatic Therapy): Two tablets twice daily; Femtrol (Enzymatic Therapy): Two capsules three times daily; Phytogen (Enzymatic Therapy): One capsule three times daily.
- For painful menstruation, try Fem-Care (Enzymatic Therapy): Two capsules three times per day, two days prior to and during menstruation.
- For congestive symptoms (water retention, breast tenderness, capillary fragility, etc.): Ginkgo Biloba Extract (Enzymatic Therapy): One capsule three times daily.
- Menstrusan (Bioforce—homeopathic)
  As directed.

PROSTATE ENLARGEMENT (BPH)

Nearly 60 percent of men between the ages of 40 and 59 years have an enlarged prostate gland, a condition referred to in the medical community as benign prostatic hyperplasia (BPH). Symptoms of BPH typically reflect obstruction of the bladder outlet: progressive urinary frequency, urgency and nighttime awakening to empty the bladder, and hesitancy and intermittency with reduced force and caliber of urine. The condition, if left untreated, will eventually obstruct the bladder outlet resulting in the retention of urine in the blood.

Diet appears to play a critical role in the development of BPH. Paramount to an effective BPH prevention and treatment plan is adequate zinc intake and absorption. Zinc has been shown to reduce the size of the prostate—as determined by rectal examination, x-ray, and endoscopy—and to reduce symptoms in the majority of patients. The clinical efficacy of zinc is probably due to its critical involvement in many aspects of hormonal metabolism.

Dietary and Lifestyle Recommendations:

- Consume a diet which focuses on whole, unprocessed foods (whole grains, legumes, vegetables, fruits, nuts, and seeds).
- Eat 1/4 cup of raw sunflower seeds or pumpkin seeds each day.
- Eliminate the intake of alcohol, caffeine, and sugar.
- Identify and control food allergies.
- Get regular exercise.
- Perform a relaxation exercise (deep breathing, meditation, prayer, visualization, etc.) for 10 to 15 minutes each day.
- Drink at least 48 ounces of water daily, but drink no fluids after 7:00 p.m.

Primary Treatment Plan:

- Doctor's Choice for Men (Enzymatic Therapy)
     One tablet three times daily.
- Doctor's Choice Antioxidant Complex (Enzymatic Therapy)
     One to two capsules three times daily.
- Doctor's Choice Flax Oil Plus (Enzymatic Therapy) or Omega Twin (Barlean's)
     One tablespoon daily.
- Super Saw Palmetto (Enzymatic Therapy)
     One capsule twice daily. (Or, Saw Palmetto Complex by Enzymatic Therapy: Two capsules twice daily).

Additional Recommendations:

- PRO-50 (Enzymatic Therapy)
     One capsule three times daily.

Comments:

Saw palmetto extract (85 to 95 percent fatty acids and sterols) at a dosage of 160 mg twice daily has been shown to be effective in roughly 90 percent of cases, making it by far the most effective agent for BPH.

PROSTATITIS

Prostatitis refers to an infection or inflammation of the prostate. Prostatitis is associated with pain during urination, fever, and a discharge from the penis. The standard medical treatment is antibiotics. With antibiotics alone the condition is typically of a chronic nature and difficult to clear. Frequent or chronic prostate infections may be a sign of low zinc levels as the prostatic fluid contains a powerful zinc-containing anti-infective substance.

Dietary and Lifestyle Recommendations:

- Consume a diet which focuses on whole, unprocessed foods (whole grains, legumes, vegetables, fruits, nuts, and seeds).
- Eat 1/4 cup of raw sunflower seeds or pumpkin seeds each day.
- Eliminate the intake of alcohol, caffeine, and sugar.
- Identify and control food allergies.
- Get regular exercise.
- Perform a relaxation exercise (deep breathing, meditation, prayer, visualization, etc.) for 10 to 15 minutes each day.
- Drink at least 48 ounces of water daily.

Primary Treatment Plan:

- Doctor's Choice for Men (Enzymatic Therapy)
      One tablet three times daily.
- Doctor's Choice Antioxidant Complex (Enzymatic Therapy)
      One to two capsules three times daily.

(continued on page 134)

Prostate cancer:
Alternative treatment strategies.

An analysis featured in the *Journal of the American Medical Association* (JAMA) revealed that treatment of localized prostate cancer, including radical prostatectomy and radiation therapy, may not be the best treatment choice.

JAMA researchers found that "watchful waiting" (i.e. no treatment) provides the patient with similar chances and an increase in quality of life when compared to radical prostatectomy and radiation. They reported "because prostatic carcinoma is a slowly growing tumor, metastasis may not occur for years after discovery of an apparently localized tumor."

Statistics show that among men with prostate cancer, approximately 60 percent have tumors localized to the prostate gland. According to the JAMA article, "prostatic carcinoma is a disease of older men, many of whom will expectedly die of other causes before developing metastatic cancer."

After considering treatment complications and quality of life, the researchers believe "the patient will experience the impact of any complications (from surgery and radiation) sooner than he will experience any benefits of treatment." Common complications of surgery and radiation include impotence and incontinence.

"If the medical community were to apply the same standards of safety and efficacy required for approval of new drugs to the use of invasive treatments for prostate cancer, it is likely that neither radical prostatectomy nor radiation therapy would be approved for this indication," reported the researchers.

The researchers concluded, "Our decision analysis shows that watchful waiting may be an appropriate alternative to invasive treatment for many men with localized prostatic carcinoma."

Julian Whitaker, M.D., a nationally-respected wellness doctor, concurs with the JAMA researchers, "Studies have determined that early treatment of small tumors of the prostate is not necessary since the majority of those patients died of other causes before the tumor could spread."

Dr. Whitaker believes in the use of a low-fat diet, standardized Saw palmetto berry extract, and close follow-up, using surgery if tumor growth begins to cause symptoms.
—JAMA, Vol. 269, No. 20, May 26, 1993; Health and Healing, Dr. Julian Whitaker, Vol. 3, No. 3, April 1993.

- Doctor's Choice Flax Oil Plus (Enzymatic Therapy) or Omega Twin (Barlean's)
    One tablespoon daily.
- PRO-50 (Enzymatic Therapy)
    One capsule three times daily.
- Aqua-Flow (Enzymatic Therapy)
    Two to four capsules four times daily (maximum one month at this high dosage).

Additional Recommendations:

If you have been on antibiotics, try Enzydophilus (Enzymatic Therapy): One capsule three times daily with meals for the first week. Thereafter, one capsule daily with a meal.

PSORIASIS

Psoriasis is a condition caused by a pile up of skin cells that have replicated too rapidly. Psoriasis is an extremely common skin disorder. Its rate of occurrence in the United States is between two and four percent of the population. A number of dietary factors appear to be responsible for psoriasis including: incomplete protein digestion; alcohol consumption; and excessive consumption of animal fats.

Dietary and Lifestyle Recommendations:

- Consume a diet which focuses on whole, unprocessed foods (whole grains, legumes, vegetables, fruits, nuts, and seeds).
- Avoid animal products with the exception of cold water fish (salmon, mackerel, herring, halibut, etc.).
- Identify and control food allergies.
- Eliminate the intake of alcohol, caffeine, and sugar.
- Get regular exercise.
- Perform a relaxation exercise (deep breathing, meditation, prayer, visualization, etc.) for 10 to 15 minutes each day.
- Drink at least 48 ounces of water daily.

Primary Treatment Plan:

- Doctor's Choice (Male/Female) (Enzymatic Therapy)
  One tablet three times daily.
- Doctor's Choice Antioxidant Complex (Enzymatic Therapy)
  Two capsules three times daily.
- Doctor's Choice Flax Oil Plus (Enzymatic Therapy) or Omega Twin (Barlean's)
  One or two tablespoons daily.
- Super Milk Thistle (Enzymatic Therapy)
  One capsule three times daily before meals.
- Mega-Zyme (Enzymatic Therapy)
  Two to four tablets twice daily between meals.
- Akne-Zyme (Enzymatic Therapy)
  One capsule twice daily.
  Note: Do not use Akne-Zyme during pregnancy (use with caution in women of child-bearing age) or when abdominal pain, nausea or vomiting are present. Also, Akne-Zyme may cause temporary gas.

Additional Recommendations:

- Simicort (Enzymatic Therapy) applied to the affected area two to three times daily.

Comments:

The components of Simicort have demonstrated an effect equal to or superior to cortisone when applied topically. Unlike cortisone creams, Simicort is without side effects.

RHEUMATOID ARTHRITIS

Rheumatoid arthritis (RA) is a chronic inflammatory condition that affects the entire body but especially the synovial membranes of the joints. It is a classic example of an "autoimmune disease," a condition in which the body's immune system attacks the body's own tissue.

In RA, the joints typically involved are the hands and feet, wrists, ankles, and knees. Somewhere between one and three percent of the population is affected; female patients outnumber males almost 3:1; and the usual age of onset is 20 to 40 years, although rheumatoid arthritis may begin at any age. The onset of rheumatoid arthritis is usually gradual, but occasionally it is quite abrupt. Fatigue, low grade fever, weakness, joint stiffness, and vague joint pain may precede the appearance of painful, swollen joints by several weeks. Several joints are usually involved in the onset, typically in a symmetrical fashion, i.e., both hands, wrists, or ankles. In about one-third of persons with RA, initial involvement is confined to one or a few joints. Involved joints will characteristically be quite warm, tender, and swollen. The skin over the joint will take on a ruddy purplish hue. As the disease progresses joint deformities result in the hands and feet. Terms used to describe these deformities include: swan neck, boutonniere, and cockup toes.

There is abundant evidence that rheumatoid arthritis is an "autoimmune" reaction, where antibodies develop against components of joint tissues. Yet what triggers this autoimmune reaction remains largely unknown. Speculation and investigation has centered around genetic susceptibility, abnormal bowel permeability, lifestyle and nutritional factors, food allergies, and microorganisms. Rheumatoid arthritis is a classic example of a multifactorial disease where there is an interesting assortment of genetic and environmental factors which contribute to the disease process. For a full discussion of all of these factors and a more comprehensive treatment plan, refer to Dr. Michael T. Murray's book on *Arthritis* (part of the *Getting Well Naturally Series*—see Appendix IV of this book).

Dietary and Lifestyle Recommendations:

- Consume a diet which focuses on whole, unprocessed foods (whole grains, legumes, vegetables, fruits, nuts, and seeds).
- Avoid animal products with the exception of cold water fish (salmon, mackerel, herring, halibut, etc.).
- Identify and control food allergies.
- Eliminate the intake of alcohol, caffeine, and sugar.
- Get regular exercise.
- Perform a relaxation exercise (deep breathing, meditation, prayer, visualization, etc.) for 10 to 15 minutes each day.
- Drink at least 48 ounces of water daily.

Primary Treatment Plan:

- Doctor's Choice (Male/Female) (Enzymatic Therapy)
    One tablet three times daily.
- Doctor's Choice Antioxidant Complex (Enzymatic Therapy)
    One to two capsules three times daily.
- Doctor's Choice Flax Oil Plus (Enzymatic Therapy) or Omega Twin (Barlean's)
    One to two tablespoons daily.
- Mega-Zyme (Enzymatic Therapy)
    Two to four tablets twice daily between meals.
- Adrenal-Cortex Complex (Enzymatic Therapy)
    One to three capsules daily.
- Curazyme (Enzymatic Therapy) or Gingerall (Enzymatic Therapy)
    Two to four tablets twice daily between meals.
- Artho-Soothe (Enzymatic Therapy)
    Apply to affected areas twice daily.

Additional Recommendations:

- If corticosteroids have been used at either high dosages or for long-term, recommend Raw Adrenal (Enzymatic Therapy) and/or Adren-Comp (Enzymatic Therapy).

Comments:

Artho-Soothe contains a pungent principle known as "capsaicin" isolated from Cayenne pepper (*Capsicum frutescens*). When applied to the skin, capsaicin is known to stimulate and then block the transmission of the pain impulse. It does this by depleting the nerves of a messenger substance called substance P (the P stands for PAIN). In addition to playing a key role in the pain impulse, substance P has also been shown to activate inflammatory mediators into joint tissues in rheumatoid arthritis.

ROSACEA

Rosacea is a chronic acne-like eruption on the face of middle-aged and older adults associated with facial flushing. The primary involvement occurs over the flush areas of the cheeks and nose. It is more common in women (3:1), but more severe in men. Many factors have been suspected of causing acne rosacea: alcoholism, menopausal flushing, local infection, B-vitamin deficiencies, and decreased secretion of digestive factors. Most cases are associated with moderate to severe seborrhea (excess flow of sebum).

Dietary and Lifestyle Recommendations:

- Eliminate all refined and/or concentrated sugars from the diet.
- Do not eat foods containing trans-fatty acids such as milk, milk products, margarine, shortening and other synthetically hydrogenated vegetable oils, as well as fried foods.
- Avoid milk and foods high in iodized salt.
- Avoid the use of greasy creams or cosmetics.
- Wash the pillowcase regularly in chemical-free (no added colors or fragrances) detergents.

Primary Treatment Plan:

- Doctor's Choice (Male/Female) (Enzymatic Therapy)
    One tablet three times daily with meals.
- Doctor's Choice Antioxidant Complex (Enzymatic Therapy)
    One capsule three times daily with meals.
- Doctor's Choice Flax Oil Plus (Enzymatic Therapy) or Omega Twin (Barlean's)
    One tablespoon daily.
- Akne-Zyme (Enzymatic Therapy)
    One capsule twice daily.
- Akne Treatment Cleanser (Enzymatic Therapy)
    Wash face or affected area with the cleanser twice daily.
- Akne Treatment Cream (Enzymatic Therapy)
    Apply one to three times daily as directed on label.
- Clear Skin (Lehning Laboratories)
    As directed on bottle.

Additional Recommendations:

- Lipozyme (Enzymatic Therapy)
    Two to four tablets 20 minutes before meals. Especially beneficial in rosacea and cystic acne.
- Lympho-Clear (Enzymatic Therapy)
    One capsule three times daily.

Comments:

Do not use Akne-Zyme during pregnancy (use with caution in women of child-bearing age) or when abdominal pain, nausea or vomiting are present. Akne-Zyme may cause temporary gas.

SCHIZOPHRENIA AND MULTIPLE PERSONALITY DISORDER

Schizophrenia is characterized by withdrawal from reality, illogical thinking patterns, delusions, and hallucinations. These features can be accompanied by varying degrees of emotional, behavioral, or intellectual disturbances. Abram Hoffer, M.D., a Canadian physician, has been a pioneer in the area of treating schizophrenia and multiple personality disorder with nutrition and nutritional supplements. Dr. Hoffer has had much clinical success treating his patients using specific vitamins and minerals. For more information contact the Canadian Schizophrenia Foundation, 16 Florence Ave., Toronto, Canada M2N 1E9.

Lifestyle and Dietary Recommendations:

- The diet must be as nutritious as possible, eliminating "junk food" completely.
- Eliminate any food allergies.

Primary Treatment Plan:

- Doctor's Choice (Male/Female) (Enzymatic Therapy)
    One tablet three times daily.

- Doctor's Choice Antioxidant Complex (Enzymatic Therapy)
    One to two capsules three times daily.
- HexaNiacin (Enzymatic Therapy)
- Vitamin B6 (any leading brand)
    500 mg daily
- Vitamin C (any leading brand)
    3 grams daily
    The optimal dose of vitamin C is the amount just below the dose which causes gas and loose bowels. This will vary; however, Dr. Hoffer recommends a minimum of three grams.
- Zinc (any leading brand)
    50 to 100 mg daily

Comments:

Additional support will be needed for individuals suffering from insomnia or depression. Refer to those sections for recommendations.

SCLERODERMA

Scleroderma refers to an autoimmune disorder that can affect many body tissues, particularly the skin, arteries, kidneys, heart, lungs, gastrointestinal tract, and joints. Symptoms are the result of abnormal collagen formation. The number and severity of the symptoms can vary drastically. The most common symptom is Raynaud's phenomena, a painful response of the hands or feet to cold exposure.

Dietary and Lifestyle Recommendations:

- Consume a diet which focuses on whole, unprocessed foods (whole grains, legumes, vegetables, fruits, nuts, and seeds).
- Avoid animal products with the exception of cold water fish (salmon, mackerel, herring, halibut, etc.).
- Identify and control food allergies.
- Eliminate the intake of alcohol, caffeine, and sugar.
- Get regular exercise.

- Perform a relaxation exercise (deep breathing, meditation, prayer, visualization, etc.) for 10 to 15 minutes each day.
- Drink at least 48 ounces of water daily.

Primary Treatment Plan:

- Doctor's Choice (Male/Female) (Enzymatic Therapy)
    One tablet three times daily.
- Doctor's Choice Antioxidant Complex (Enzymatic Therapy)
    One to two capsules three times daily.
- Doctor's Choice Flax Oil Plus (Enzymatic Therapy) or Omega Twin (Barlean's)
    One to two tablespoons daily.
- Mega-Zyme (Enzymatic Therapy)
    Two to four tablets twice daily between meals.
- Adrenal-Cortex Complex (Enzymatic Therapy)
    One to three capsules daily.
- Curazyme (Enzymatic Therapy)
    Two to four tablets twice daily between meals.
- Cellu-Var (Enzymatic Therapy)
    Two capsules twice daily.

Additional Recommendations:

If corticosteroids have been used at either high dosages or long-term, recommend Raw Adrenal (Enzymatic Therapy) and/or Adren-Comp (Enzymatic Therapy).

Comments:

The standardized extract of *Centella asiatica* contained in Cellu-Var has been tested in several trials in the treatment of scleroderma (including systemic sclerosis). In addition to decreased skin hardening, patients have noticed a lessening of joint pain and improved finger motility. Presumably, the positive therapeutic response is a result of *Centella's* balancing effect on connective tissue, thereby preventing the excessive collagen synthesis observed in scleroderma.

SINUS INFECTION

An acute sinus infection is characterized by nasal congestion and discharge fever, chills, and frontal headache, and pain, tenderness, redness, and swelling over the involved sinus. A chronic infection may produce no symptoms other than mild postnasal discharge, a musty odor, or a nonproductive cough.

The most common predisposing factor in acute bacterial sinusitis is viral upper respiratory tract infection (e.g., the common cold). Allergies and other factors which interfere with normal protective mechanisms may precede the viral infection and, therefore, are also likely predisposing factors. Any factor which induces swelling and fluid retention of the mucous membranes of the sinuses may cause blockage of drainage. In this scenario, bacterial overgrowth occurs.

In chronic sinus infections (sinusitis) an allergic background is commonly present, and in 25 percent of chronic maxillary sinusitis, there is an underlying dental infection.

Dietary and Lifestyle Recommendations:

• Avoid cigarette smoke and other respiratory irritants.
• Rest.
• Drink at least 48 ounces of water daily.
• Avoid sugar and dairy products.

Primary Treatment Plan: (Acute Treatment)

• ThymuPlex (Enzymatic Therapy)
     Two tablets twice daily.
• Vitamin C (any leading brand)
     500 to 1,000 mg every waking hour or to bowel tolerance.
• Hydrastine (Enzymatic Therapy)
     Four capsules three times daily with glass of water.
• Air-Power (Enzymatic Therapy)
     Follow dosage recommendation on bottle.
• Sinus Formula (Lehning Laboratories)
     20 drops in three ounces of water every two to three hours, three to five times per day.

Additional Recommendations:

- Sinusan (Bioforce—homeopathic)
  As directed.
- The following can be performed twice daily: Apply a heating pad, hot water bottle, hot compress, or mustard poultice to the sinus area for up to twenty minutes. A mustard poultice is made by mixing one part dry mustard with three parts flour and adding enough water to make a paste. After the hot pack, have the individual perform postural drainage by lying with the top half of the body off the bed using the forearms as support. The position should be assumed for a five to 15 minute period while attempting to blow nose, cough and expectorate into a basin or newspaper on the floor.

SPORTS INJURIES

(see BURSITIS AND TENDONITIS)

STRESS

The damaging effects of stress on our health have been well documented. Recognizing and coping with stress will be very important to your overall health. Ultimately, the success of any stress management program will depend on its ability to improve an individual's immediate and long-term response to stress. Dealing with stress will require:

1. A comprehensive stress management plan that includes time management and new coping methods.
2. Calming the mind and body with relaxation techniques and bodywork.
3. Paying attention to diet by reducing or eliminating caffeine and alcohol, creating healthful eating habits, and eliminating food allergies.

4. Regular exercise.

5. Nutritional supplement support.

Lifestyle and Dietary Recommendations:

- Practice relaxation techniques such as meditation, yoga, etc.
- Get massages, or other forms of bodywork as necessary.
- Exercise regularly; however, avoid exercising before bedtime.
- Eat fresh fruits and vegetables and drink plenty of water.

Primary Treatment Plan:

- Doctor's Choice (Male/Female) (Enzymatic Therapy)
    One tablet three times daily.
- Stress End (Enzymatic Therapy)
    One to three capsules daily
    Contains important B vitamins, minerals and herbs to help your body cope with stressful situations.
- Adrenal Extract (Enzymatic Therapy)
    By supporting the adrenal glands, your body will be able to deal with stress appropriately without allowing the stress to negatively affect your health.
- Ginseng (Enzymatic Therapy)
    If you are under mild to moderate stress, you can try Siberian ginseng; however, if you are under a great deal of stress, recovering from a long-standing illness, or have ever taken corticosteroids like prednisone, you will want to use Panax ginseng. Visit your local health food store for ginseng choices. Be sure to use a product that is standardized.

Additional Recommendations:

- Anti-Anxiety (Lehning Laboratories)
    This homeopathic formula will help calm the nerves and should be used for individuals feeling anxiety associated with their stress.
- Vitamin C (any leading brand)
    Extra vitamin C will not only help your body cope with stress it will also stimulate your immune system, which becomes weakened during times of stress.

- Adaptogen (Rainbow Light)
    Contains siberian ginseng for adrenal support—as directed.
- Nervosan (Bioforce—homeopathic)
    As directed.
- Liquid Kalm (Natrol)
    As directed.

Comments:

According to nutritionist, Ann Louise Gittleman, if you're "stressed out," you need to support your adrenal glands with vitamins, minerals, and the proper nutrients found in a healthy diet. By nourishing your body, you will be more apt to handle stressful situations. Key conditions that Gittleman feels contribute to stress are candida, parasites, and/or digestive disorders. For more information on any of those subjects, refer to that particular section.

To determine your stress level, complete the stress questionnaire on page 146.

STROKES

(see CEREBROVASCULAR INSUFFICIENCY)

SORE THROAT and TONSILLITIS

(see INFECTION)

Stress:
Rate your stress level...

A popular method of rating stress levels is the social readjustment rating scale. Various events are numerically rated according to their potential for causing disease. A total of 200 or more units in one year is considered to be predictive of the likelihood of getting a serious disease.

Rank	Life event	Value Score
1	Death of spouse	100
2	Divorce	73
3	Marital separation	65
4	Jail term	63
5	Death of a close family member	63
6	Personal injury or illness	53
7	Marriage	50
8	Fired at work	47
9	Marital reconciliation	45
10	Retirement	45
11	Change in health of family member	44
12	Pregnancy	40
13	Sex difficulties	39
14	Gain of a new family member	39
15	Business adjustment	39
16	Change in a financial state	38
17	Death of a close friend	37
18	Change to different line of work	36
19	Change in number of arguments with spouse	35
20	Large mortgage	31
21	Foreclosure of mortgage or loan	30

22	Change in responsibilities at work	29
23	Son or daughter leaving home	29
24	Trouble with in-laws	29
25	Outstanding personal achievement	28
26	Spouse begins or stops work	26
27	Begin or end school	26
28	Change in living conditions	25
29	Revision of personal habits	24
30	Trouble with boss	23
31	Change in work hours or conditions	20
32	Change in residence	20
33	Change in schools	20
34	Change in recreation	19
35	Change in church activities	19
36	Change in social activities	18
37	Small mortgage	17
38	Change in sleeping habits	16
39	Change in number of family get-togethers	15
40	Change in eating habits	15
41	Vacation	13
42	Christmas	12
43	Minor violations of the law	11

TOTAL

SURGERY PREPARATION AND RECOVERY

Any surgical procedure requires special nutritional attention. Major surgeries, especially abdominal surgery, can benefit by natural measures designed to reduce inflammation and swelling while promoting proper wound healing. These measures will not only improve recovery, but also help prevent adhesion and excessive scar formation.

Surgery Preparation

- Begin at least two weeks prior to surgery.
- Doctor's Choice (Male/Female) (Enzymatic Therapy)
    One tablet three times daily.
- Doctor's Choice Antioxidant Complex (Enzymatic Therapy)
    One to two capsules three times daily.
- Doctor's Choice Flax Oil Plus (Enzymatic Therapy) or Omega Twin (Barlean's)
    One tablespoon daily.
- Cellu-Var (Enzymatic Therapy)
    Two capsules twice daily.
- Vitamin C (any leading brand)
    1,000 to 3,000 mg daily in divided dosages.
- Grape Seed (PCO) Phytosome (Enzymatic Therapy)
    One capsule three times daily.

Recovery

- All of the above, plus Bromelain Plus (Enzymatic Therapy)
    Two tablets twice daily between meals.
- Continue for at least one month after surgery.

Comments:

Adhering to a healthful diet before and after surgery will also be important.

ULCER

An ulcer usually refers to a peptic ulcer, a term which is used to refer to a group of ulcerative disorders of the upper gastrointestinal tract. The major forms of peptic ulcer are chronic duodenal and gastric (stomach) ulcer. Although duodenal and gastric ulcerations occur at different locations, they appear to be the result of similar mechanisms. Specifically, the development of a duodenal or gastric ulcer is generally thought to be the result of pepsin and stomach acids damaging the lining of the duodenum or stomach. Normally there are enough protective factors to prevent the ulcer formation, however, when there is a decrease in the integrity of these protective factors, ulceration occurs.

Although symptoms of a peptic ulcer may be absent or quite vague, most often peptic ulcers are associated with abdominal discomfort noted 45 to 60 minutes after meals or during the night. In the typical case, the pain is described as gnawing, burning, cramp-like, or aching, or as "heartburn." Eating or using antacids usually results in great relief.

NOTE: Individuals with any symptoms of a peptic ulcer need competent medical care. Peptic ulcer complications such as hemorrhage, perforation, and obstruction represent medical emergencies that require immediate hospitalization. Patients with peptic ulcer should be monitored by a physician, even if following the natural approaches discussed below.

The natural approach to peptic ulcers is to first identify, and then eliminate or reduce all factors which can contribute to the development of peptic ulcers: food allergy, low-fiber diet, cigarette smoking, stress, and drugs such as aspirin and other nonsteroidal analgesics. Once the causative factors have been controlled or eliminated, the focus is directed at healing the ulcers and promoting tissue resistance.

Dietary and Lifestyle Recommendations:

- Consume a diet that focuses on whole, unprocessed foods (whole grains, legumes, vegetables, fruites, nuts, and seeds).
- Eliminate milk and other dairy products.
- Get regular exercise.
- Drink at least 48 ounces of water daily.

Primary Treatment Plan:

- Doctor's Choice (appropriate formula) (Enzymatic Therapy)
    One tablet three times daily.
- Doctor's Choice Antioxidant Complex (Enzymatic Therapy)
    One to two capsules three times daily.
- Doctor's Choice Flax Oil Plus (Enzymatic Therapy) or Omega Twin (Barlean's)
    One tablespoon daily.
- DGL (Enzymatic Therapy) or DGL Power (Nature's Herbs)
    Two to four chewable tablets 20 minutes before meals.

Additional Recommendations:

- GastroSoothe (Enzymatic Therapy) in place of the DGL
    Two to four chewable tablets 20 minutes before meals.
- Robert's Formula (Enzymatic Therapy or Gaia Herbs, Inc.)
    As directed.

VARICOSE VEINS

Varicose veins affect nearly 50 percent of middle-aged adults. The veins just under the skin of the legs are the veins most commonly affected, due to the tremendous strain that standing has on these veins. When an individual stands for long periods of time, the pressure exerted against the vein can increase up to ten times. Hence, individuals with occupations that require long periods of standing are at greatest risk for developing varicose veins.

Women are affected about four times as frequently as men; obese individuals have a much greater risk; and the risk increases with age due to loss of tissue tone, loss of muscle mass, and weakening of the walls of the veins. Pregnancy may also lead to the development of varicose veins, as pregnancy increases venous pressure in the legs.

Dietary and Lifestyle Recommendations:

- Consume a diet which focuses on whole, unprocessed foods (whole grains, legumes, vegetables, fruits, nuts, and seeds).
- Get regular exercise.
- Drink at least 48 ounces of water daily.

Primary Treatment Plan:

- Doctor's Choice (appropriate formula) (Enzymatic Therapy)
    One tablet three times daily.
- Doctor's Choice Antioxidant Complex (Enzymatic Therapy)
    One to two capsules three times daily.
- Doctor's Choice Flax Oil Plus (Enzymatic Therapy) or Omega Twin (Barlean's)
    One tablespoon daily.
- Cellu-Var (Enzymatic Therapy)
    Two capsules twice daily.
- Aorta-Glycan (Enzymatic Therapy)
    One capsule twice daily.

Additional Recommendations:

- Cellu-Var Cream (Enzymatic Therapy)
    Apply twice daily over affected areas.
- Varisan (Bioforce—homeopathic)
    As directed.

Comments:

In general, varicose veins pose little harm if the involved vein is small and near the surface. These types of varicose veins are, however, cosmetically unappealing. Although significant symptoms are not common, the legs may feel heavy, tight, and tired. Larger varicose veins and a more serious form of varicose vein that involves obstruction and valve defects of the deeper veins of the leg need medical attention.

Weight Loss

Maintaining an optimum weight provides many health benefits. Science has now confirmed that being overweight is linked to serious illnesses such as cancer and heart disease. Unfortunately, many people continue to have difficulty losing weight.

Long-lasting weight loss can only be accomplished using a comprehensive approach that includes making a commitment to healthy lifestyles.

Lifestyle and Dietary Recommendations:

- Exercise on a regular basis (work up to 30 to 40 minutes, three to four times per week).
- Eat a diet made up of fresh fruits and vegetables, while limiting high-fat foods and avoiding sugar and sweets.

Primary Treatment Plan:

- Hypo-Aid (Enzymatic Therapy)
    To help curb sugar cravings, this product contains nutrients that will improve sugar and carbohydrate metabolism.
- Slimming Formula (Lehning Laboratories)
    This homeopathic formula will help you control your appetite while stimulating a healthy metabolism.
- CitriLean (Enzymatic Therapy)
    This supplement contains CitriMax™, a natural compound extracted from the fruit rind of *Garcinia cambogia*, and ChromeMate® brand chromium, which helps convert fat into muscle. It does not contain caffeine, ephedrine, or other stimulants.

Additional Recommendations:

- Escalation (Enzymatic Therapy)
    If energy is a problem, this thermogenic formula will help speed up the metabolism. Not suitable for pregnant women or people with high blood pressure, heart disease, thyroid disease, diabetes, or difficulty in urination due to enlargement of the prostate. In addition, ephedrine products should not be used by patients taking antihypertensive or antidepressant drugs.
- Sambu internal cleansing and weight loss program (Flora)
    3-day or 10-day programs are available.

Comments:

While nutritional supplements can provide important support to individuals trying to lose weight, nothing can replace a healthy diet and regular exercise. Lasting weight loss will require a commitment to making important lifestyle changes. Exercise is a key component to any successful weight loss program. Some type of regular, physical activity should be performed a minimum of three times a week for 30 to 40 minutes each. If you are presently inactive, see your doctor before beginning any regular exercise program.

Because individual dietary and weight loss needs vary, refer to Ann Louise Gittleman's book, *Your Body Knows Best*, listed in Appendix IV of this book.

Appendix I

Quick Reference Guide to Nutrients

Nutrient	Importance	Deficiency Symptoms
Vitamin A	Necessary for growth and repair of body tissues. Important to health of the eyes. Fights bacteria and infection. Maintains healthy epithelial tissue. Aids in bone and teeth formation.	Night blindness. Rough, dry, scaly skin. Increased susceptibility to infections. Frequent fatigue, insomnia, depression. Loss of smell and appetite. Lusterless hair. Brittle nails. Inflamed eyelids.
Vitamin B complex	Necessary for carbohydrate, fat, and protein metabolism. Helps functioning of the nervous system. Helps maintain muscle tone in the gastrointestinal tract. Maintains health of skin, hair, eyes, mouth, and liver.	Dry, rough, cracked skin. Acne. Dull, dry, or grey hair. Fatigue. Poor appetite. Gastrointestinal tract disorders.
Vitamin B1 (Thiamine)	Necessary for carbohydrate metabolism. Helps maintain healthy nervous system. Stabilizes growth and good muscle tone. Stabilizes the appetite.	Gastrointestinal problems. Fatigue. Loss of appetite. Nerve disorders. Heart disorders. Poor impulse control.

Nutrient	Importance	Deficiency Symptoms
Vitamin B2 (Riboflavin)	Necessary for carbohydrate, fat, and protein metabolism. Aids in formation of antibodies and red blood cells. Maintains cell respiration.	Eye problems. Cracks and sores in mouth. Dermatitis. Retarded growth. Digestive disturbances.
Niacin (B3, Nicotinic acid, Niacinamide)	Necessary for carbohydrate, fat, and protein metabolism. Helps maintain health of skin, tongue, and digestive system.	Dermatitis. Nervous disorders. Headaches. Insomnia. Bad breath. Digestive disturbances.
Pantothenic Acid (Vitamin B5)	Aids in formation of some fats. Participates in the release of energy from carbohydrates, fats, and proteins. Aids in the utilization of some vitamins. Improves body's resistance to stress.	Sore mouth and gums. Vomiting. Restlessness. Increased susceptibility to infection. Gastrointestinal disturbances. Depression. Fatigue.
Vitamin B6 (Pyridoxine)	Necessary for carbohydrate, fat, and protein metabolism. Aids in formation of antibodies. Helps maintain balance of sodium and phosphorus.	Anemia. Mouth disorders. Nervousness. Muscular weakness. Dermatitis. Dandruff. Water retention.

Nutrient	Importance	Deficiency Symptoms
Vitamin B12	Essential for normal formation of blood cells. Necessary for carbohydrate, fat, and protein metabolism. Maintains healthy nervous system.	Pernicious anemia. Brain damage. Nervousness. Neuritis.
Folic Acid (Folacin)	Important in red blood cell formation. Aids metabolism of proteins. Necessary for growth and division of body cells.	Poor growth. Gastrointestinal disorders. Anemia. Poor memory.
Vitamin C	Maintains collagen. Helps heal wounds, scar tissue, and fractures. Gives strength to blood vessels. May provide resistance to infections. Aids in absorption of iron.	Bleeding gums. Swollen or painful joints. Slow-healing wounds and fractures. Bruising. Nosebleeds. Impaired digestion.
Vitamin D	Improves absorption and utilization of calcium and phosphorus required for bone formation. Maintains stable nervous system and normal heart action.	Poor bone and tooth formation. Softening of bones and teeth. Inadequate absorption of calcium. Retention of phosphorus in kidney.

Nutrient	Importance	Deficiency Symptoms
Vitamin E	Protects fat-soluble vitamins. Protects red blood cells. Essential in cellular respiration. Inhibits coagulation of blood by preventing blood clots.	Rupture of red blood cells. Muscular wasting. Abnormal fat deposits in muscles.
Vitamin K	Necessary for formation of prothrombin. Needed for blood coagulation.	Lack of prothrombin, increasing the tendency to hemorrhage.
Bioflavonoids (Vitamin P)	Help increase strength of capillaries.	Tendency to bleed and bruise easily.
Essential fatty acids	Important for respiration of vital organs. Help maintain resilience and lubrication of cells. Help regulate blood coagulation. Essential for normal glandular activity.	Brittle, lusterless hair. Brittle nails. Dandruff. Diarrhea. Varicose veins.
Calcium	Sustains development and maintenance of strong bones and teeth. Assists normal blood clotting, muscle action, nerve function, and heart function.	Tetany. Softening bones. Back and leg pain. Brittle bones. Insomnia. Irritability. Depression.

Nutrient	Importance	Deficiency Symptoms
Chromium	Stimulates enzymes in metabolism of energy and synthesis of fatty acids, cholesterol, and protein. Increases effectiveness of insulin.	Depressed growth rate. Glucose intolerance in diabetics. Atherosclerosis.
Copper	Aids in formation of red blood cells. Part of many enzymes. Works with vitamin C to form elastin.	General weakness. Impaired respiration. Skin sores.
Iodide	Essential part of the hormone thyroxine. Necessary for the prevention of goiter. Regulates production of energy and rate of metabolism. Promotes growth.	Enlarged thyroid gland. Dry skin and hair. Loss of physical and mental vigor. Cretinism in children born to iodine-deficient mothers.
Iron	Necessary for hemoglobin and myoglobin formation. Helps in protein metabolism. Promotes growth.	Weakness. Paleness of skin. Constipation. Anemia.
Magnesium	Acts as a catalyst in the utilization of carbohydrates, fats, protein, calcium, phosphorus, and possibly potassium.	Nervousness. Muscular excitability. Tremors. Depression.

Nutrient	Importance	Deficiency Symptoms
Manganese	Enzyme activator. Plays a part in carbohydrate and fat production. Necessary for normal skeletal development. Maintains sex-hormone production.	Paralysis. Convulsions. Dizziness. Ataxia. Blindness and deafness in infants. Diabetes. Loss of hearing.
Phosphorus	Works with calcium to build bones and teeth. Utilizes carbohydrates, fats and proteins. Stimulates muscular contractions.	Loss of weight and appetite. Irregular breathing. Pyorrhea. Nervous disorders. Fatigue.
Potassium	Works to control activity of the heart muscles, nervous system, and kidneys.	Poor reflexes. Respiratory failure. Cardiac arrest. Nervous disorders. Constipation. Irregular pulse. Insomnia.
Selenium	Works with vitamin E. Preserves tissue elasticity.	Premature aging.
Sulfur	Part of amino acids. Essential for formation of body tissues. Part of the B vitamins. Plays a part in tissue respiration. Necessary for collagen synthesis.	Possibly sluggishness and fatigue.

Nutrient	Importance	Deficiency Symptoms
Zinc	Component of insulin and male reproductive fluid. Aids in digestion and metabolism of phosphorus. Aids in healing process.	Retarded growth. Delayed sexual maturity. Prolonged healing of wounds. Stretch marks. Irregular menses. Diabetes. Loss of taste and appetite.

Appendix II

Quick Reference Guide to Herbal Extracts

Herb		Key Uses
Aloe Vera	Topical—	Wound healing Sunburn Minor skin irritations
	Oral—	Constipation Peptic ulcers Immune system enhancement
Angelica species		Menopausal symptoms Premenstrual syndrome Allergies Smooth muscle spasm
Bilberry		Diabetic retinopathy Macular degeneration Cataract Glaucoma Varicose veins
Bromelain		Inflammation Sports injuries Respiratory tract infections Painful menstruation Adjunct in cancer therapy
Cat's claw (*Una de Gato*)		Immune disorders HIV/AIDS
Cayenne pepper		Antioxidant support

Herb		Key Uses
Cayenne pepper (cont.)		Atherosclerosis
		Asthma
		Pain disorders
		Diabetic neuropathy
		Cluster headaches
		Arthritis
		Psoriasis
Coleus forskohlii		Eczema
		Asthma
		Psoriasis
		Angina
		High blood pressure
Dandelion	Root—	Liver tonic
	Leaves—	Diuretic
		Weight loss aid
Echinacea		Common cold
		Infections
		Low immune status
		Cancer
Ephedra		Asthma
		Hay fever
		Common cold
		Weight loss aid
Feverfew		Migraine headaches
		Fever
		Inflammation
Garlic		Cancer prevention
		Diabetes
		High blood pressure and high cholesterol

Herb	Key Uses
Garlic (cont.)	Infection
Ginger	Nausea and vomiting Motion sickness Arthritis Migraine headaches
Gingko biloba	Cerebral vascular insufficiency (insufficient blood flow to the brain) Dementia Depression Impotence Inner ear dysfunction (vertigo, tinnitus, etc.) Multiple sclerosis Neuralgia and neuropathy Peripheral vascular insufficiency (intermittent claudication, Raynaud's disease, etc.) Premenstrual syndrome Retinopathy (macular degeneration, diabetic retinopathy, etc.) Vascular fragility
Goldenseal	Infections of mucous membranes Parasitic infections of the gastrointest- inal tract Inflammation of the gallbladder Cirrhosis of the liver
Gotu kola	Cellulite Wound healing Varicose veins Scleroderma

Herb	Key Uses
Grape seed extract	Antioxidant supplementation Atherosclerosis prevention Capillary fragility and easy bruising Diabetes Retinopathy (macular degeneration and diabetic retinopathy) Varicose veins Wound healing
Green tea	Antioxidant supplementation Cancer prevention
Gugulipid	High cholesterol levels High triglyceride levels
Hawthorn	Angina Atherosclerosis Congestive heart failure High blood pressure
Kava	Anxiety Depression Insomnia
LaPacho (Pau d' Arco)	Infections Cancer Candida albicans
Licorice	Viral infections including the common cold, viral hepatitis, AIDS Inflammation Menstrual and menopausal disorders
Deglycyrrhizinated licorice (DGL)	Peptic Ulcers Canker sores

Herb		Key Uses
Topical glycyrrhetinic acid		Herpes
		Eczema
		Psoriasis
Lobelia		Smoking deterrent
		Asthma
		Bronchitis
		Pneumonia
Milk thistle		Liver disorders
		Hepatitis
		Cirrhosis of the liver
		Gallstones
		Psoriasis
Mistletoe		Cancer
		Impaired thymus gland activity
		Immune system enhancement
		High blood pressure
Onion		Infections
		Elevated cholesterol levels
		High blood pressure
		Diabetes
Panax Ginseng		Fatigue
		Recovery from illness
		Stress
		Diabetes
Peppermint	Oral—	Gallstones
		Irritable bowel syndrome
		Common cold
	Topical—	Musculoskeletal pain

Herb	Key Uses
Pygeum	Benign prostatic hyperplasia
	Prostatitis
	Male infertility
	Impotence
St. John's wort	Depression
	Sleep disorders
	Viral infections
Sarsaparilla	Psoriasis
	Eczema
	General tonic
Saw palmetto	Benign prostatic hyperplasia
Siberian ginseng	Stress and fatigue
	Atherosclerosis
	Impaired kidney function
Tea tree oil	Topical antiseptic
	Fungal nail infections
	Acne
	Vaginal infections
Turmeric (Curcumin)	Antioxidant
	Cancer prevention and treatment
	Gallstones
	Inflammatory conditions
	Irritable bowel syndrome
	Liver disorders
Uva ursi	Urinary tract infection
	As a mild diuretic
Valerian	Insomnia
	Stress and anxiety

Appendix III

Health Counselor Index

Following is a list of articles that have appeared in past issues of *Health Counselor* magazine. For more information on ordering back issues, call 1-800-477-2995.

Acne . . . . March/April 1991
Acne/All natural treatment plan. . . . . Oct/Nov 1995
Acne, cystic . . . . Volume 4, No. 4
Acne/Tea tree oil and zinc . . . . Volume 4, No. 6
Addictions/Breaking free. Feb/March 1995
Aggressive behavior/Nutrients . . . . Volume 5, No. 4
Aging. . . . . Special '91 Edition
Aging/Dietary allowances . . . . Volume 4, No. 5
Aging/Nutrients prevent disease. . . . . Volume 5, No. 3
Aging/Selenium . . . . Volume 4, No. 4
Aging/Vitamin B12 . . . . Volume 4, No. 4
AIDS and HIV . . . . June/July 1995
AIDS/Aloe vera. . . . . Volume 5, No. 2
AIDS/Natural healing . . . . May/June 1991
AIDS/Immune dysfunction . . . . Volume 4, No. 4
AIDS/St. John's wort . . . . May/June 1991
AIDS/Update . . . . Volume 5, No. 4
AIDS/Update . . . . June/July 1994
Alcoholism/Nutritional treatment. . . . . Volume 5, No. 1
Alcoholism/Vitamin E . . . . March/April 1991
Allergies, food . . . . Volume 4, No. 6
Allergies/Homeopathic formulas . . . . Aug/Sept 1994
Allergies/Natural relief . . . . Volume 4, No. 3

Allergies/Putting an end to . . . . Aug/Sept 1995

Allergies/Vitamin C. . . . . Volume 4, No. 6

Allergy elimination diet . . . . Volume 4, No. 6

Alzheimer's disease/Amino acids. . . . . Volume 4, No. 5

Alzheimer's disease . . . . April/May 1994

Alzheimer's disease . . . . Special '91 Edition

Alzheimer's/selenium, zinc, primrose oil . . . . Volume 4, No. 3

Anemia/Liquid liver extract . . . . Feb/March 1994

Angina pectoris/Antioxidants. Volume 4, No. 3

Anxiety . . . . Volume 4, No. 5

Anxiety/Healing with homeopathy. . . . . Dec/Jan 1996

Anxiety/Kava . . . . Dec/Jan 1995

Anxiety and depression. . . . . Oct/Nov 1995

Anxiety and panic attacks . . . . Dec/Jan 1995

Arthritis/Boron . . . . Volume 5, No. 4

Arthritis/Effective treatment for. . . . . Dec/Jan 1995

Arthritis/Glucosamine. . . . . Aug/Sept 1995

Arthritis/Glucosamine sulphate . . . . Aug/Sept 1994

Arthritis/Treatment breakthrough . . . . Volume 5, No. 2

Asthma . . . . Volume 4, No. 3

Asthma/Hope for sufferers. . . . . Volume 5, No. 4

Asthma/Nutritional therapies. Volume 4, No. 4

Atherosclerosis/Vitamin B6 . . . . Volume 4, No. 4

Atherosclerosis/Hawthorn . . . . Volume 5, No. 1

Athletic injuries/children. . . . . April/May 1995

Attention Deficit Hyperactivity Disorder . . . . Feb/March 1994

Attention Deficit Disorder/Thyroid. . . . . June/July 1994

Autism. . . . . June/July 1994

Back Pain/Relief for. . . . . June/July 1995

Backaches . . . . Aug/Sept 1994

Birth defects/Folate. . . . . Feb/March 1994

Bladder condition. . . . . Volume 5, No. 2

Bladder infections/Chronic . . . . Volume 5, No. 1

Bladder infections/Cystitis. . . . . April/May 1994

Bladder infections/Recurring . . . . April/May 1994

Bladder problems. . . . . Volume 5, No. 4

Blood pressure . . . . Aug/Sept 1995

Blood pressure/Maitake mushroom . . . . April/May 1995

Blood pressure/Omega-3 fish oil . . . . March/Apr 1991

Blood pressure/Potassium depletion. . . . . March/Apr 1991

Blood pressure/Calcium in children. . . . . Volume 4, No. 3

Blood pressure/Controlling . . . . Volume 5, No. 1

Blood pressure/Hawthorn . . . . Volume 5, No. 1

Blood pressure/Potassium . . . . Volume 4, No. 5

Bone density/Spinal and calcium. . . . . Volume 4, No. 2

Bone health . . . . Volume 4, No. 2

Bone spurs. . . . . Volume 4, No. 3

Bone spurs. . . . . Feb/March 1994

Bone strength/Walking . . . . May/June 1991

Brain function/Amino acid tyrosine . . . . Special '91 Edition

Brain function/L-tyrosine and L-tryptophan . . . . June/July 1995

Brain power. . . . . Oct/Nov 1995

Breast milk study . . . . June/July 1995

Breathing/Nutrients. . . . . May/June 1991

Bruising. . . . . Oct/Nov 1994

Burn scars . . . . Volume 4, No. 5

B Vitamin deficiencies/Resemble leukemia. . . . . Volume 4, No. 6

Calcium absorption/Fiber . . . . Volume 4, No. 2

Cancer. . . . . Aug/Sept 1995

Cancer/Alert for women . . . . Volume 4, No. 5

Cancer/Beta carotene and vitamin C . . . . Special '91 Edition

Cancer/Dietary sugar . . . . Aug/Sept 1994

Cancer/EFAs. . . . . Feb/March 1995
Cancer/Fighting foods . . . . Volume 5, No. 2
Cancer/Fish oil . . . . Aug/Sept 1994
Cancer/Folic acid deficiencies. . . . . Volume 4, No. 3
Cancer/Garlic. . . . . June/July 1994
Cancer/Maitake mushroom . . . . April/May 1995
Cancer/Nutrition. . . . . Volume 4, No. 6
Cancer/Psychological stress. . . . . Volume 5. No. 5
Cancer/Prevention . . . . Volume 5, No. 4
Cancer/Selenium . . . . Volume 4, No. 4
Cancer/Selenium . . . . Aug/Sept 1994
Cancer/Shark liver oil . . . . Dec/Jan 1995
Cancer/Shark Cartilage . . . . Feb/March 1994
Cancer/Vitamin B . . . . Mar/April 1991
Cancer/Vitamin C. . . . . Volume 5, No. 1
Cancer/Vitamins . . . . April/May 1994
Cancer in women/Folic acid . . . . Volume 4, No. 5
Cancer treatment/Centers . . . . Volume 4, No. 4
Cancer treatment plan/Karolyn Gazella . . . . Aug/Sept 1995
Cancer treatment/Psychological intervention . . . . Dec/Jan 1995
Cancer treatment/Unconventional . . . . Volume 5, No. 3
Cancer Treatment Center of America . . . . Oct/Nov 1995
Cancer, breast . . . . Oct/Nov 1994
Cancer, breast . . . . Feb/March 1995
Cancer, breast/Estrogen. . . . . Oct/Nov 1995
Cancer, breast/Fiber . . . . Volume 4, No. 3
Cancer, childhood/Vitamin K. . . . . Feb/March 1994
Cancer, colon/Vitamin D and calcium. . . . . Volume 4, No. 3
Cancer, colon/Prevention . . . . Volume 5, No. 5
Cancer/Protection with ginseng. . . . . Volume 4, No. 6
Cancer, prostate/Fiber. . . . . May/June 1991

Cancer/Risk reduction with flaxseed . . . . Volume 4, No. 2

Cancer, skin/Signs of. . . . . Volume 4, No. 4

Cancer/The war on. . . . . Volume 4, No. 4

Cancer/The war on. . . . . Volume 4, No. 5

Cancer/The war on. . . . . Volume 4, No. 6

Candida/Controlling naturally . . . . June/July 1995

Canker sores . . . . Volume 4, No. 5

Canker sores/Natural relief . . . . Volume 4, No. 5

Cardiovascular system/Garlic . . . . Feb/March 1995

Carpal tunnel syndrome/Vitamin B6 . . . . Volume 4, No. 4

Carpal tunnel syndrome/Supplements . . . . Aug/Sept 1994

Cataracts/Prevention of. . . . . Volume 5, No. 2

Cell growth/Zinc. . . . . Volume 4, No. 3

Cellulite/Herbal support for. . . . . Mar/April 1991

Chalazions. . . . . Feb/March 1995

Chemical sensitivity . . . . April/May 1994

Cholesterol. . . . . Volume 4, No. 3

Cholesterol. . . . . Aug/Sept 1995

Cholesterol/Ginger . . . . Volume 4, No. 4

Cholesterol/Good and bad . . . . Special '91 Edition

Cholesterol/Gugulipid. . . . . Dec/Jan 1996

Cholesterol/Magnesium . . . . Volume 4, No. 6

Cholesterol/Psyllium. . . . . Dec/Jan 1995

Cholesterol level reduction/Psyllium . . . . Special '91 Edition

Chronic fatigue syndrome. . . . . Dec/Jan 1995

Chronic fatigue syndrome/Low magnesium . . . . Special '91 Edition

Chronic intestinal cystitis/Supplements for . . . . Mar/Apr 1991

Cirrhosis/Lecithin . . . . May/June 1991

Cirrhosis/Silymarin . . . . Mar/April 1991

Cold and flu/Homeopathy, the smart choice. . . . . Oct/Nov 1994

Cold symptoms/Zinc. . . . . Volume 5, No. 1

Cold/Common . . . . Volume 5, No. 1
Colds/Medications ineffective . . . . Volume 5, No. 5
Colds/Vitamin C . . . . Volume 4, No. 6
Colds/Vitamin E . . . . Special '91 Edition
Cold sores and herpes outbreaks . . . . Feb/March 1995
Colon cancer/Vitamin D and calcium . . . . Volume 4, No. 3
Connective tissue . . . . Volume 4, No. 6
Connective tissue disorders . . . . June/July 1994
Cravings/Iron deficiency . . . . Volume 4, No. 3
Cystic acne . . . . Volume 4, No. 4
Cystic fibrosis/Vitamin E . . . . Mar/April 1991
Cystitis . . . . April/May 1995
Cystitis/Bladder infections . . . . April/May 1994
Dental health . . . . Oct/Nov 1994
Depression and anxiety/Relief . . . . Oct/Nov 1995
Depression/Calcium . . . . June/July 995
Depression/St. John's wort . . . . April/June 1995
Depression/St. John's wort . . . . Aug/Sept 1995
Dermatitis/Evening primrose . . . . Volume 4, No. 4
Dermatitis/Vitamin E . . . . Aug/Sept 1994
Detoxification . . . . Mar/April 1991
Detoxification/Nutrients for . . . . Volume 5, No. 2
DiabetesSpecial '91 Edition Diabetes . . . . Aug/Sept 1995
Diabetes/Common spices . . . . Volume 4, No. 5
Diabetes/Natural alternatives . . . . April/May 1995
Digestion/Healthy . . . . Volume 4, No. 6
Digestion/Pancreatic enzymes . . . . Volume 5, No. 4
Disease/Enzymes fighting . . . . Oct/Nov 1994
Dizziness . . . . Volume 4, No. 2
Dizziness . . . . June/July 1995
Ear infections/Alternatives to surgery . . . . Volume 4, No. 5

Ear infections/Children . . . . Feb/March 1995
Ear infections/Children April/May1995
Ear infections/Recurrent in children . . . . Dec/Jan 1996
Ears/lumps under . . . . Volume 4, No.3
Ears/Ringing . . . . Feb/March 1994
Ears/Ringing . . . . Oct/Nov 1994
Eczema/Herbal tea . . . . Volume 5, No. 2
Endometriosis . . . . Dec/Jan 1996
Energy . . . . April/May 1995
Esophageal distress . . . . Feb/March 1994
Estrogen replacement therapy . . . . Volume 4, No. 2
Estrogen replacement therapy . . . . Oct/Nov 1995
Eyes/Dry and vitamins . . . . Volume 4, No. 3
Eyes/Damage from computer use . . . . Oct/Nov 1994
Eye conditions/Chalzion . . . . Feb/March 1995
Eyesight/Protecting . . . . Special '91 Edition
Eyesight/Supporting . . . . Special '91 Edition
Fatigue/Potassium . . . . Special '91 Edition
Fertility, male/Vitamin C . . . . Volume 4, No. 4
Fibrocystic breast disease . . . . Aug/Sept 1994
Fibrocystic breast disease . . . . Aug/Sept 1995
Fibromyalgia . . . . Special '91 Edition
Fibromyalgia . . . . June/July 1995
Flatulence . . . . June/July 1994
Flu and cold/Echinacea . . . . Oct/Nov 1994
Flu and cold/Homeopathy . . . . Oct/Nov 1994
Food allergies . . . . Volume 4, No. 6
Gallbladder removal/Digestive problems . . . . April/May 1995
Gallstones/Prevention . . . . Volume 4, No. 4
Gastritis . . . . Volume 5, No.1
Glandular therapy . . . . Volume 5, No. 3

Gout . . . . Volume 5, No. 1

Gums/Pockets of bacteria . . . . Volume 5, No. 2

Hair loss/Legs. . . . . Feb/March 1994

Hair, skin, nails . . . . June/July 1995

Hay fever . . . . Volume 4, No. 3

Headaches/Chronic . . . . Volume 5, No. 2

Health/Seven principles . . . . Volume 5, No. 1

Health dangers/Insect repellent . . . . Volume 4, No. 5

Hearing/Preventing loss . . . . Special '91 Edition

Heart/Hawthorn . . . . Volume 5, No. 1

Heart/Iron . . . . Volume 5, No. 1

Heart/L-Arginine. . . . . Feb/March 1995

Heart/Magnesium . . . . Volume 4, No. 6

Heart/Potassium . . . . Special '91 Edition

Heart/Potassium . . . . Aug/Sept 1994

Heart attack/Earlobe crease. . . . . Special '91 Edition

Heart attacks/High blood pressure drugs . . . . Dec/Jan 1996

Heart attacks/Magnesium . . . . Volume 4, No. 5

Heart disease/Answers to . . . . Volume 4, No. 3

Heart disease/Antioxidants . . . . Oct/Nov 1994

Heart disease/Antioxidants . . . . Feb/March 1995

Heart disease/Eradicating . . . . Feb/March 1994

Heart disease/Eradicating with nutrients. . . . . April/May 1994

Heart disease/Copper deficiency . . . . Volume 4, No. 5

Heart disease/Is it reversible?. May/June 1991

Heart disease/Magnesium . . . . Dec/Jan 1995

Heart disease/Vitamin C . . . . Volume 5, No. 1

Heart disease/Vitamin E . . . . Volume 5, No. 4

Heart disease/Vitamin E . . . . Oct/Nov 1995

Heart health/Antioxidants . . . . Special '91 Edition

Heart health/Beta carotene . . . . May/June 1991

Heart health/Coenzyme Q10 . . . . Volume 4, No. 3

Heart medications/Harmful . . . . Volume 5, No. 3

Heart rate/Vitamin C and athletes . . . . Volume 4, No. 3

Hepatitis/Naomi Judd's healing journey . . . . Dec/Jan 1996

Herpes and cold sore outbreaks . . . . Dec/Jan 1995

Herpes virus/Strengthen immune system . . . . June/July 1995

Hiatal hernia . . . . Feb/March 1994

High blood pressure/Cholesterol . . . . Aug/Sept 1995

HIV/Chinese medication . . . . April/May 1994

HIV and AIDS/Alternative medicine . . . . June/July 1995

Homeopathic medicine . . . . Aug/Sept 1994

Homeopathy/Effective . . . . Volume 5, No. 3

Homeopathy . . . . Volume 5, No. 2

Hormonal imbalance . . . . Volume 5, No. 1

Hyperactivity/Food additives . . . . June/July 1995

Hypertension/Nutrients for . . . . Volume 5, No. 3

Immune system . . . . May/June 1991

Immune system . . . . Volume 5, No. 1

Immune responses/Zinc deficiencies . . . . Volume 4, No. 2

Immunity/Exercise . . . . May/June 1991

Immunity/Zinc . . . . Volume 4, No. 3

Impotence . . . . June/July 1994

Infants/Algae improves formula . . . . Volume 4, No. 2

Infections/Copper . . . . Mar/April 1991

Infections/St. John's wort . . . . Feb/March 1994

Infertility, male . . . . Dec/Jan 1996

Infertility/Chinese herbs . . . . Dec/Jan 1995

Inflammation/Curcumin . . . . Special '91 Edition

Inflammation/Enzymes . . . . June/July 1994

Inflammation/Pancreatic enzymes . . . . Volume 5, No. 4

Injury/Children in athletics . . . . April/May 1995

Injury/Prevention and treatment. . . . . June/July 1995

Insomnia . . . . Feb/March 1994

Intermittent claudication (leg cramps) . . . . Volume 4, No. 5

Interstitial pulmonary fibrosis . . . . Dec/Jan 1995

Intestinal flora growth. . . . . Mar/April 1991

Iron deficiency anemia/Infants. . . . . Volume 4, No. 3

Irritable bowel syndrome (IBS). . . . . Dec/Jan 1995

Kidney disease/OTC drugs . . . . Oct/Nov 1995

Kidney health/Spirulina. . . . . May/June 1991

Kidney stones/Calcium citrate . . . . Mar/April 1991

Kidney stones/Prevention . . . . Volume 4, No. 5

Kidney stones/Vitamin C. . . . . Aug/Sept 1994

Knees/Cracking. . . . . Volume 4, No. 5

Leg cramps/Pregnancy . . . . Volume 4, No. 2

Leg cramps (intermittent claudication) . . . . Volume 4, No. 5

Lichen spinulosa/Treatment. Volume 5, No. 1

Lipofuscin . . . . Volume 5, No. 1

Liquid liver extract . . . . Feb/March 1994

Liver extracts . . . . Volume 5, No. 4

Liver function/Proper support . . . . Volume 5, No. 4

Liver function/Proper support . . . . Feb/March 1995

Liver/Elevated enzymes. . . . . Volume 5, No. 4

Liver/Silymarin. . . . . Mar/April 1991

Longevity/Antioxidants . . . . Special '91 Edition

Lupus. . . . . Volume 4, No. 4

Lyme disease . . . . May/June 1991

Lyme disease . . . . June/July 1994

Macular degeneration/Zinc. Special '91 Edition

Macular degeneration. . . . . Volume 4, No. 5

Male infertility/Treating. . . . . Dec/Jan 1996

Measles/Vitamin A . . . . Volume 5, No. 2

Menopause . . . . Volume 5, No. 2

Menopause/Estrogen replacement . . . . Volume 4, No. 5

Menopause/Ginseng. . . . . Volume 4, No. 6

Menopause/Natural therapy . . . . Dec/Jan 1995

Menopause/Natural therapy . . . . Special '91 Edition

Menopause/Phytoestrogens . . . . Volume 5, No. 4

Menorrhagia (heavy menstrual bleeding) . . . . Volume 4, No. 6

Menstrual discharge/Bioflavonoids. . . . . Special '91 Edition

Menstrual problems/Herbs for . . . . Oct/Nov 1994

Mental acuity/Iron and zinc . . . . Special '91 Edition

Mental function/Zinc . . . . Volume 4, No. 5

Mental health/Exercise . . . . Oct/Nov 1995

Mental health/Nutrition. . . . . Volume 4, No. 6

Mental wisdom . . . . Feb/March 1994

Migraine, PMS/Magnesium . . . . Volume 4, No. 2

Migraine/Relief. . . . . Aug/Sept 1995

Migraine/Feverfew . . . . Mar/April 1991

Migraine/Feverfew . . . . April/May 1995

Morning sickness/Ginger. . . . . Volume 4, No. 4

Mosquito bites . . . . Oct/Nov 1994

Motion sickness/Ginger root . . . . Mar/April 1991

Motion sickness/Ginger. . . . . Volume 4, No. 4

Multiple sclerosis . . . . Aug/Sept 1994

Muscle damage/Antioxidants. . . . . Volume 5, No. 1

Muscle growth/Vitamin E . . . . Volume 5, No. 2

Muscle spasms/Amino acids . . . . Special '91 Edition

Narcolepsy. . . . . Volume 4, No. 3

Narcolepsy/L-tyrosine. . . . . Mar/April 1991

Nausea/Ginger. . . . . Volume 4, No. 4

Nervous system/Vitamin B12. . . . . Special '91 Edition

NTD (neurol tube defects)/Folic acid . . . . Volume 4, No. 2

NTD (neurol tube defects)/Folic acid . . . . Volume 5, No. 2
Obsessive-compulsive disorder . . . . Volume 4, No. 2
Obsessive-compulsive disorder . . . . Volume 4, No. 3
Osteoarthritis . . . . Aug/Sept 1995
Osteoarthritis/Ayurvedic medicine . . . . Feb/March 1995
Osteoarthritis/Glucosamine . . . . Dec/Jan 1995
Osteoarthritis/Natural relief . . . . June/July 1994
Osteoporosis . . . . Volume 4, No. 2
Osteoporosis/Magnesium . . . . Volume 4, No. 2
Osteoporosis/Preventing and reversing . . . . Dec/Jan 1996
Osteoporosis/Thyroid hormone . . . . May/June 1991
Osteoporosis/Vitamin K . . . . Volume 5, No. 4
Pain relief/Amino acids . . . . Special '91 Edition
Pain relief/Glucosamine sulfate . . . . Aug/Sept 1994
Pancreatic enzymes . . . . Volume 5, No. 4
Panic attacks . . . . Volume 4, No. 5
Panic attacks and anxiety/Natural relief . . . . Dec/Jan 1995
Parasites . . . . April/May 1995
Parkinson's disease . . . . Feb/March 1994
Parkinson's disease/Vitamins . . . . Volume 4, No. 3
Periodontal concerns . . . . Volume 5, No. 2
Plaque . . . . April/May 1994
Platelet count/Low . . . . Volume 4, No. 5
PMS/Calcium . . . . Volume 4, No. 2
PMS/Migraines and magnesium . . . . Volume 4, No. 2
PMS/Multi-nutrient supplements . . . . Volume 4, No. 2
PMS/Natural relief . . . . Volume 4, No. 2
PMS/Relief . . . . Aug/Sept 1995
PMS/Strength or weakness . . . . Oct/Nov 1995
PMS/Vitamin E . . . . Special '91 Edition
Pregnancy/Alcohol . . . . Volume 4, No. 2

Pregnancy/Caffeine. . . . . Aug/Sept 1995
Pregnancy/Calcium. . . . . Volume 4, No. 2
Pregnancy/Exercise. . . . . Dec/Jan 1996
Pregnancy/Fitness. . . . . Volume 4, No. 2
Pregnancy/Leg cramps . . . . Volume 4, No. 2
Pregnancy/Morning sickness and ginger. . . . . Volume 4, No. 4
Pregnancy/Nutrition . . . . Volume 4, No. 2
Pregnancy/Preparing. . . . . Oct/Nov 1995
Pregnancy/Vitamin B6 and nausea. . . . . Volume 4, No. 2
Pregnancy/What to avoid . . . . Volume 4, No. 2
Pregnancy/Zinc . . . . Volume 4, No. 3
Prostate . . . . Aug/Sept 1994
Prostate/Enlarged . . . . Volume 5, No. 4
Prostate/Enlarged . . . . Aug/Sept 1994
Prostate/Enlarged . . . . Aug/Sept 1995
Prostate/Inflamed . . . . Volume 5, No. 1
Prostate/Saw palmetto. . . . . Aug/Sept 1995
Prostate/Saw palmetto. . . . . April/May 1995
Psoriasis/Cayenne. . . . . June/July 1994
Psoriasis/Herbs. . . . . April/May 1995
Psoriasis/Natural therapies . . . . Volume 4, No. 2
Pycnogenol/Protection . . . . Feb/March 1994
Rashes/Skin . . . . Volume 5, No.1
Raynaud's syndrome. . . . . Feb/March 1995
Red blood cells/Too many. . . . . Volume 4, No. 2
Reproductive health/Vitamin B12 . . . . Special '91 Edition
Rheumatoid arthritis. . . . . Volume 4, No. 3
Rheumatoid arthritis/Tumeric. . . . . Volume 4, No. 3
Rheumatoid arthritis/Treatment . . . . Aug/Sept 1994
Rupture wort (Herniari glabra). . . . . Volume 4, No. 4
Schizophrenia/Orthomolecular approach. . . . . April/May 1994

Sebaceous Cysts. . . . . Volume 4, No. 3

Senility . . . . Special '91 Edition

Sexual health/Zinc . . . . Volume 4, No. 3

Sinus/Relief . . . . Aug/Sept 1995

Skin rashes. . . . . Volume 5, No.1

Skin/Save it from harm . . . . Volume 4, No. 4

Skin/Summertime care . . . . Volume 4, No. 6

Skin/Vitamins. . . . . Special '91 Edition

Smell, loss of/Zinc . . . . Volume 4, No. 3

Spleen . . . . Volume 4, No. 5

Spleen/Damage . . . . Oct/Nov 1995

Stress/Attitude. . . . . June/July 1995

Stress/Cancer . . . . Volume 5, No. 5

Stroke/Potassium. . . . . Special '91 Edition

Stroke/Recovery and Vitamin A . . . . Volume 5, No. 1

Taste, loss of/Zinc. . . . . Volume 4, No. 3

Teeth/Healthy with fluorine. April/May 1995

Teeth/Healthy with molybdenum. . . . . April/May 1995

Thyroid/Iodine . . . . Feb/March 1995

Tinea versicolor (yeast infection of the skin). . . . . Volume 4, No. 6

TMJ/Nutritional support . . . . May/June 1991

Tourette syndrome . . . . Aug/Sept 1995

Ulcers/Natural healing . . . . Volume 4, No. 6

Ulcers/Natural treatment. . . . . Volume 5, No. 2

Ulcers, peptic/Natural approach . . . . Dec/Jan 1996

Urinary infections/Cranberries. . . . . Feb/March 1995

Vaginal itching/Bladder infections . . . . April/May 1994

Vertigo (dizziness) . . . . June/July 1995

Vision loss/Nutrients. . . . . Volume 4, No. 5

Vitiligo (loss of skin pigment) . . . . Volume 4, No. 4

Weight gain/Healthy; muscle not fat . . . . Volume 4, No. 5

Weight loss . . . . Volume 5, No. 1
Weight loss/Bariatrics . . . . Feb/March 1995
Weight loss/Bariatrics . . . . Dec/Jan 1995
Weight loss/Citrimax and chromium . . . . Oct/Nov 1995
Weight loss/Natural aids . . . . Volume 5, No. 3
Weight loss/Thermogenesis . . . . Volume 5, No. 2
Weight loss/Thermogenesis . . . . June/July 1994
Weight management/Homeopathy . . . . June/July 1995
Wounds/Aloe . . . . Aug/Sept 1995
Yeast infection . . . . Volume 4, No. 6

To order any of these back issues call 1-800-477-2995 in the United States, 1-888-292-2229 in Canada (MasterCard, VISA, Discover and American Express accepted) or send a check or money order ($4 each up to five magazines, $3 each for six or more magazines) to:

IMPAKT Communications
Attn: *Health Counselor* Back Issues
P.O. Box 12496
Green Bay, WI 54307-2496

Please specify which back issues you are ordering and where you would like them sent.

Appendix IV

Here is a list of other fine books published or distributed by IMPAKT Communications:

Alternative Medicine: The Definitive Guide published by the Burton
      Goldberg Group
      Hardcover, 1068 pages, $55.00

Beating Cancer with Nutrition by Patrick Quillin, Ph.D.
      Paperback, 254 pages, $16.95

Breast Cancer by Steve Austin, N.D. and Cathy Hitchcock, M.S.W.
      Paperback, 336 pages, $18.95

Dr. Whitaker's Guide to Natural Healing by Julian Whitaker, M.D.
      Hardcover, 417 pages, $17.95

Encyclopedia of Natural Medicine by Michael T. Murray, N.D.
      Paperback, 622 pages, $21.95

Flavor Without Fat by best-selling author Jan McBarron, M.D.
      Paperback, 312 pages, $17.95

Ginger: Common Spice & Wonder Drug by Paul Schulick
      Paperback, 166 pages, $11.95

Getting Well Naturally Series by Michael T. Murray, N.D.
      Paperback, $10.95 each, all six for $60.00

      Arthritis, 158 pages
      Chronic Fatigue Syndrome, 196 pages
      Diabetes and Hypoglycemia, 164 pages
      Male Sexual Vitality, 150 pages
      Menopause, 182 pages
      Stress, Anxiety, and Insomnia, 178 pages

Healing Power of Herbs by Michael T. Murray, N.D.
Paperback, 410 pages, $17.95

Help Yourself: The Beginner's Guide to Natural Medicine
by Karolyn A. Gazella
Paperback, 134 pages, $10.95

Natural Alternatives to Over-the Counter and Prescription Drugs by
Michael T. Murray, N.D.
Hardcover, 383 pages, $30.00

Natural Alternatives to Prozac by Michael T. Murray, N.D.
Hardcover, 192 pages, $22.00

Preventing and Reversing Osteoporosis by Alan R. Gaby, M.D.
Paperback, 304 pages, $16.95

Questions and Answers on Family Health— The Alternative Approach by
Jan de Vries, M.D.
Paperback, 280 pages, $ 5.95

Seven Keys to Vibrant Health by Terry Lemerond
Paperback, 113 pages, $12.95

Your Body Knows Best by Ann Louise Gittleman and James Templeton
with Candelora Versace
Paperback, 288 pages, $23.00

All prices include the shipping and handling costs.
If you are interested in ordering any of these books, call IMPAKT
Communications at 1-800-477-2995.

The following informational booklets are also available through IMPAKT Communications, Inc.:

• *Melissa Extract: The Natural Herbal Remedy for Herpes* by Jan de Vries

    48 pages, $3.95

• *Remifemin: Herbal Relief for Menopausal Symptoms* by Frank Murray

    48 pages, $3.95

• *Enjoying Childbearing to the Fullest* by Carl Jones

    24 pages, $3.00

• *Natural Healing for Parasites* by Ann Louise Gittleman

    12 pages, $2.00

Quantity discounts for the booklets listed above are available. To order one or more of the booklets, call 1-800-477-2995 or send a check or money order to IMPAKT Communications, Inc., P.O. Box 12496, Green Bay, WI 54307-2496. MasterCard, VISA, or American Express orders must be a minimum of $3.95 per order.

Glossary

Acupuncture

This procedure uses needles to penetrate and stimulate specific points throughout the body. The purpose of acupuncture is to restore normal body function and renew the body's energetic balance.

Amino acids

Amino acids are considered the building blocks of protein. There are 22 separate amino acids: 13 can be manufactured in the body and the other 9 are available through dietary protein. Nutritional supplements often contain certain amino acids. Specific amino acids work closely with specific body functions. For example, L-tryptophan is an essential amino acid that influences brain function. Amino acids are available within dietary supplement formulations or as separate products.

Antioxidant

A compound/nutrient which prevents free-radical and oxidative damage.

Ayurvedic medicine

Originating in India, ayurvedic medicine is an ancient form of treatment that involves diet, detoxification, exercise, herbal medicine and meditation. Ayurvedic medicine is effective for the treatment of a wide variety of chronic health conditions.

Biofeedback

This type of training teaches the patient how to consciously control their autonomic (involuntary) nervous system by using biofeedback devices which sound a tone when changes in pulse, blood pressure, brain waves, and muscle contractions occur. Biofeedback training is most commonly used to alleviate stress, migraine headaches, asthma, and high blood pressure.

Chelation therapy

Chelation therapy is a medical process that uses an intravenous solution to remove heavy metals and toxins from the blood. It is commonly used to reverse atherosclerosis and as an alternative to bypass surgery and angioplasty. Chelation therapy has also been shown to reduce high blood pressure and help reverse age-related degenerative diseases.

Free radical

Highly reactive molecules that bind to and detroy cells. Free radical toxins can be found in the air we breathe, the water we drink, and the foods we eat.

Glandular therapy

Glandular therapy uses extracts as an important form of medicine. Glandular therapy believes that like heals like. For example, if your liver needs therapeutic support, you may benefit from eating beef liver. Modern glandular therapy, however, uses concentrated glandular extracts, which contain active hormones and enzymes. Glands commonly used in extracts include the pituitary, thyroid, thymus, pancreas, and adrenal. Other organs, such as heart, spleen, liver, etc., can also be used as glandular extracts. Glandular extracts can be sold separately or as part of a dietary supplement formulation.

Guided imagery

This type of meditation capitalizes on the power of the mind by creating mental pictures that help stimulate a positive physical response. It is commonly used to help stimulate the immune system, reduce stress, and slow heart rate.

Herbal medicine

Having an extensive history of usage throughout the world, herbal medicine uses plant substances as medicine. Research has shown herbal medicines to be effective in a wide range of conditions.

Homeopathy

Homeopathic medicine uses minute traces of a medicinal substance to stimulate the healing processes of the body in order to restore health and normal body function. Homeopathy is used extensively in England, Europe, Mexico, and India.

Hypnotherapy

This is a method used to tap into a person's unconscious mind to help facilitate the treatment of a variety of conditions including depression, stress, anxiety, obesity, and eating disorders.

Naturopathy

This is a system of medicine based upon natural principles of health and a respect for the healing power of nature. Naturopathy, also known as naturopathic medicine, utilizes therapies such as diet, herbal medicine, hydrotherapy, lifestyle counseling, acupuncture, and homeopathy to help the body heal itself.

Osteopathy

Osteopathic physicians use body manipulation, physical, medicinal, and surgical techniques to restore good health and balance within their patients. This is known as osteopathy, which is designed to remove any internal or external abnormalities. It is recognized as a standard method or system of medical and surgical care.

Standardized botanical extracts

A botanical extract is an herb that is used for medicinal purposes. It is estimated that about 25 percent of all prescription drugs in the United States contain active constituents obtained from plants. Botanical extracts have a long history of use as herbal medicines. Standardization is a scientific technique used to ensure quality and consistency among botanical products. Botanical extracts standardized for a specific active constituent ensure each and every capsule has the same potency to provide the user with consistent results.

Sidebar Index

To find the page number of a particular condition, refer to the contents. Following is a listing of sidebars featured throughout this book.

ARTICLE TITLE	PAGE
AIDS Update: High nutrient intake slows disease development.	11
Healing Addictions: Prevention is the best medicine of all!	15
The Ritalin Rage: How is this drug affecting our children?	28
Comprehensive cancer treatment: The mind plays an important role in recovery.	39
Candida Questionnaire: Are your health concerns yeast-connected?	42
The Sugar Blues: Determine your status with this self-appraisal.	67
Magnesium plays important role in heart health.	21
Glucosamine sulfate vs. NAG.	118
Osteoporosis: Are you at risk?	122
Parkinson's Disease: Nutrient treatment results quite promising.	126
Prostate Cancer: Alternative treatment strategies.	133
Rate your stress level	146

Order *Health Counselor* magazine and receive a FREE book...

Health Counselor will provide you with the most accurate, up-to-date holistic healthcare information you need to make healthy choices. Healthcare experts from throughout the United States and Canada share their knowledge about vitamins, minerals, herbs, and other natural health alternatives. Get the information you need to make appropriate health choices—subscribe to *Health Counselor* magazine today.

One-year (six information-packed issues) = $18 (U.S.) $29 (Canada)

Two-year (12 information-packed issues) = $32 (U.S.) $55 (Canada)

To subscribe send a check or money order with the completed form below to:

IMPAKT Communications, Inc.
P.O. Box 12496
Green Bay, WI 54307-2496

MasterCard, VISA, and American Express Orders can call 1-800-477-2995 (must mention free book offer when placing order by phone).

Order a subscription and receive a FREE *Dr. Whitaker's Guide to Natural Healing* by Julian Whitaker, M.D. This hardcover, 417-page book provides important information on nearly 100 specific health conditions. It's a $23 value and it's yours FREE when you subscribe to *Health Counselor.*

Send my *Health Counselor* subscription and my FREE book to:

Name

Address

City/State/Zip

Phone

Method of payment (circle one): MasterCard, VISA, American Express, Check/Money Order

Card No.   Exp. date

Signature